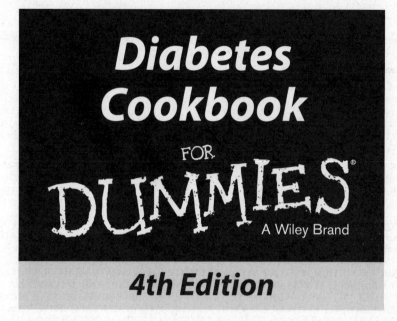

Diabetes Cookbook FOR DUMMIES®
A Wiley Brand

4th Edition

by Alan L. Rubin, MD,
with Cait James, MS

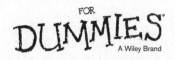

Diabetes Cookbook For Dummies,® 4th Edition

Published by: **John Wiley & Sons, Inc.,** 111 River Street, Hoboken, NJ 07030-5774, www.wiley.com

Copyright © 2015 by John Wiley & Sons, Inc., Hoboken, New Jersey

Published simultaneously in Canada

For general information on our other products and services, please contact our Customer Care Department within the U.S. at 877-762-2974, outside the U.S. at 317-572-3993, or fax 317-572-4002. For technical support, please visit www.wiley.com/techsupport.

Wiley publishes in a variety of print and electronic formats and by print-on-demand. Some material included with standard print versions of this book may not be included in e-books or in print-on-demand. If this book refers to media such as a CD or DVD that is not included in the version you purchased, you may download this material at http://booksupport.wiley.com. For more information about Wiley products, visit www.wiley.com.

Library of Congress Control Number: 2014945061

ISBN 978-1-118-94426-4 (pbk); ISBN 978-1-118-94427-1 (ebk); ISBN 978-1-118-94428-8 (ebk)

Manufactured in the United States of America

10 9 8 7 6 5 4 3 2 1

Contents at a Glance

Recipes at a Glance

Entrees 173

Table of Contents

Introduction

People with diabetes can eat great food! You can follow a diabetic diet at home or anywhere you travel and still enjoy a five-star meal. You just have to know how to cook it or where to go to get it. And that's where this book comes in. Here, we show you how to prepare great foods in your own home and give you a guide to eating out.

Is diet important for a person with diabetes? Do salmon swim upstream? The Diabetes Control and Complications Trials showed that a good diabetic diet could lower the hemoglobin A1c, a test of overall blood glucose control, by over 1 percent. That much improvement will result in a reduction of complications of diabetes such as eye disease, nerve disease, and kidney disease by 25 percent or more. The progression of complications that have already started to occur can be significantly slowed.

Of course, there's much more to managing diabetes than diet alone. In this book, you can discover the place of diet in a complete program of diabetes care.

About This Book

This edition of *Diabetes Cookbook For Dummies* features many new recipes based on the Mediterranean diet. Many new studies have shown that people who follow a Mediterranean diet have a lower incidence of diabetes. And if they already have diabetes, a Mediterranean diet makes it easier to control. (We explain the Mediterranean diet in Chapter 2.)

You wouldn't read a cookbook from cover to cover, and this book is no exception to that rule. There's no reason to read about setting up your kitchen if you simply want a place to eat in New York where you can find healthy nutrition for your diabetes. You may want to read the first few chapters to get an overview of the place of diet in your overall diabetes management, but if you just need a great entree for tonight's supper or a great restaurant wherever you are, go right to that information. The book is written to be understood no matter where you find yourself in it.

Within this book, you may note that some web addresses break across two lines of text. If you're reading this book in print and want to visit one of these web pages, simply key in the web address exactly as it's noted in the text, pretending as though the line break doesn't exist. If you're reading this as an e-book, you've got it easy — just click the web address to be taken directly to the web page.

Here are a few guidelines to keep in mind about the recipes:

- ✔ All butter is unsalted. Margarine is not a suitable substitute for butter, because of the difference in flavor and nutritional value. Butter is a natural product, while margarine is man-made and contains trans fatty acids.

- ✔ All eggs are large.

- ✔ All flour is all-purpose unless otherwise specified.

- ✔ All milk is lowfat unless otherwise specified.

- ✔ All onions are yellow unless otherwise specified.

- ✔ All pepper is freshly ground black pepper unless otherwise specified.

- ✔ All salt is table salt unless otherwise specified.

- ✔ All mentions of Splenda refer to the regular sugar substitute unless Splenda for Baking is specified.

- ✔ All dry ingredient measurements are level — use a dry ingredient measuring cup, fill it to the top, and scrape it even with a straight object, such as the flat side of a knife.

- ✔ All temperatures are Fahrenheit. (See Appendix C for information about converting temperatures to Celsius.)

- ☺ If you need or want vegetarian recipes, scan the list of "Recipes in This Chapter" on the first page of each chapter in Part II. A little tomato, rather than a triangle, in front of the name of a recipe marks that recipe as vegetarian. (See the tomato to the left of this paragraph.)

This isn't a complete book about diagnosing and treating diabetes and its complications. Check out *Diabetes For Dummies,* 4th Edition (Wiley), if you need diagnosis and treatment information.

Foolish Assumptions

The book assumes that you've done some cooking, you're familiar with the right knife to use to slice an onion without cutting your finger, and you can tell one pot from another. This book also assumes that you have an interest in diabetes prevention or management — whether for yourself or a loved one.

Icons Used in This Book

The icons in this book are like bookmarks, pointing out information that we think is especially important. Here are the icons used in this book:

We use this icon whenever Dr. Rubin tells a story about his patients.

Whenever we want to emphasize the importance of the current information to your nutritional plan, we use this icon.

When you see the Remember icon, pay special attention because the information is essential.

This icon flags situations when you should see your doctor (for example, if your blood glucose level is too high or you need a particular test done).

This helpful icon marks important information that can save you time and energy.

Watch for this icon; it warns about potential problems (for example, the possible results if you don't treat a condition).

Beyond the Book

In addition to the material in the print or e-book you're reading right now, this product also comes with some access-anywhere goodies on the web. Check out the free Cheat Sheet at www.dummies.com/cheatsheet/diabetescookbook for tips on finding your ideal weight, menu terms to look for and avoid when you're eating out, and how to improve your diet.

You can also find several online articles at www.dummies.com/extras/diabetescookbook. Whether you're interested in exercise, the Mediterranean lifestyle, or myths about diabetes, head online to read more.

Where to Go from Here

Where you go from here depends on your immediate needs. If you want an introduction to the place of nutrition in diabetes management, start with Chapter 1. If you're hungry and you want some lunch, go to Part II. If you're about to travel or eat out, head for Part III. At any time, the Part of Tens can provide useful tips for healthy eating. Finally, the appendixes help you cook for yourself or choose a restaurant. Feel free to jump around, but take the time to go through Part II so that you realize that diabetes and great food are not mutually exclusive.

Part I
Flourishing with Diabetes

In this part . . .

- ✔ Understand diabetes and its possible consequences.
- ✔ See effect food has on your diabetes.
- ✔ Select food based on your weight goal.
- ✔ Enjoy the healthy foods you choose.
- ✔ Make the supermarket your ally.

Chapter 1

What It Means to Flourish with Diabetes

Since the third edition of *Diabetes Cookbook For Dummies* came out, there have been a number of studies that indicate that a Mediterranean diet may be beneficial in the prevention and treatment of diabetes. In this new edition, we provide some of the rationale for that type of diet. You will also find 25 new recipes from some of the finest Mediterranean restaurants in the country. In this chapter, you get the latest information about what diabetes means, how diabetes is diagnosed, and the things you need to do to thrive with diabetes. Don't waste another minute. Get started right away.

Recognizing Diabetes

With so much diabetes around these days, you may think that recognizing it should be easy. The truth is that it's not easy, because diabetes is defined by blood tests. You can't just look at someone and know the level of glucose — blood sugar — in his or her blood.

Defining diabetes

The level of glucose that means you have diabetes is as follows:

- ✔ A *casual* blood glucose of 200 milligrams per deciliter (mg/dl) or more at any time of day or night, along with symptoms such as fatigue, frequent urination and thirst, slow healing of skin, urinary infections, and vaginal itching in women. A normal casual blood glucose should be between 70 and 139 mg/dl.

- ✔ A *fasting* blood glucose of 126 mg/dl or more after no food for at least eight hours. A normal fasting blood glucose should be less than 100 mg/dl.

- ✔ A blood glucose of 200 mg/dl or greater two hours after consuming 75 grams of glucose.

A diagnosis of diabetes requires at least two abnormal levels on two different occasions. Don't accept a lifelong diagnosis of diabetes on the basis of a single test.

A fasting blood glucose between 100 and 125 mg/dl or casual blood glucose between 140 and 199 mg/dl is *prediabetes*. See Dr. Rubin's book *Prediabetes For Dummies* (Wiley). Most people with prediabetes will develop diabetes within ten years. Although people with prediabetes don't usually develop small blood vessel complications of diabetes like blindness, kidney failure, and nerve damage, they're more prone to large vessel disease like heart attacks and strokes, so you want to get that level of glucose down. Sixty million people in the United States have prediabetes.

The American Diabetes Association has added a new criteria for the definition of diabetes, based around a person's A1C number. A1C is a measure of the average blood glucose for the last 60 to 90 days. If the A1C is equal to or greater than 6.5 percent, the person is considered to have diabetes.

Categorizing diabetes

The following list describes the three main types of diabetes:

- ✔ **Type 1 diabetes:** This used to be called *juvenile diabetes* or *insulin-dependent diabetes*. It mostly begins in childhood and results from the body's self-destruction of its own pancreas. The pancreas is an organ of the body that sits behind the stomach and makes insulin, the chemical or "hormone" that gets glucose into cells where it can be used. You can't live without insulin, so people with type 1 diabetes must take insulin shots. Of the 26 million Americans with diabetes, about 10 percent have type 1.

✔ **Type 2 diabetes:** Once called *adult-onset diabetes,* type 2 used to begin around the age of 40, but it is occurring more often in children, many of whom are getting heavier and heavier and exercising less and less. The problem in type 2 diabetes is not a total lack of insulin, as occurs in type 1, but a resistance to the insulin, so that the glucose still doesn't get into cells but remains in the blood.

✔ **Gestational diabetes:** This type of diabetes is like type 2 diabetes but occurs in women during pregnancy, when a lot of chemicals in the mother's blood oppose the action of insulin. About 4 percent of all pregnancies are complicated by gestational diabetes. If the mother isn't treated to lower the blood glucose, the glucose gets into the baby's bloodstream. The baby produces plenty of insulin and begins to store the excess glucose as fat in all the wrong places. If this happens, the baby may be larger than usual and therefore may be hard to deliver. When the baby is born, he is cut off from the large sugar supply but is still making lots of insulin, so his blood glucose can drop severely after birth. The mother is at risk of gestational diabetes in later pregnancies and of type 2 diabetes as she gets older. Women should be screened for gestational diabetes at 24 to 28 weeks of the pregnancy.

✔ **Other types:** A small group of people with diabetes suffer from one of these much less common varieties of diabetes:

- Latent autoimmune diabetes on adults (LADA), which has characteristics of both type 1 and type 2 diabetes
- Genetic defects of the beta cell, which makes insulin
- Medications that affect insulin action like cortisol or prednisone
- Diseases or conditions that damage the pancreas like pancreatitis or cystic fibrosis
- Genetic defects in insulin action

Knowing the consequences of diabetes

If your blood glucose isn't controlled — that is, kept between 70 and 139 mg/dl after eating or under 100 mg/dl fasting — damage can occur to your body. The damage can be divided into three categories: irritations, short-term complications, and long-term complications.

Irritations

Irritations are mild and reversible but still unpleasant results of high blood glucose levels. The levels aren't so high that the person is in immediate life-threatening danger. The most important of these irritations are the following:

✔ Blurred vision

✔ Fatigue

✔ Frequent urination and thirst

✔ Genital itching, especially in females

✔ Gum and urinary tract infections

✔ Obesity

✔ Slow healing of the skin

Short-term complications

These complications can be very serious and lead to death if not treated. They're associated with very high levels of blood glucose — in the 400s and above. The three main short-term complications are the following:

✔ **Ketoacidosis:** This complication is found mostly in type 1 diabetes. It is a severe acid condition of the blood that results from lack of insulin, the hormone that is missing. The patient becomes very sick and will die if not treated with large volumes of fluids and large amounts of insulin. After the situation is reversed, however, the patient is fine.

✔ **Hyperosmolar syndrome:** This condition is often seen in neglected older people. Their blood glucose rises due to severe dehydration and the fact that the kidneys of the older population can't get rid of glucose the way younger kidneys can. The blood becomes like thick syrup. The person can die if large amounts of fluids aren't restored. They don't need that much insulin to recover. After the condition is reversed, these people can return to a normal state.

✔ **Hypoglycemia or low blood glucose:** This complication happens when the patient is on a drug like insulin or a pill that drives the glucose down but isn't getting enough food or is getting too much exercise. After it falls below 70 mg/dl, the patient begins to feel bad. Typical symptoms include sweating, rapid heartbeat, hunger, nervousness, confusion, and coma if the low glucose is prolonged. Glucose by mouth, or by venous injection if the person is unconscious, is the usual treatment. This complication usually causes no permanent damage.

Long-term complications

These problems occur after ten or more years of poorly controlled diabetes or, in the case of the macrovascular complications, after years of prediabetes or diabetes. They have a substantial impact on quality of life. After these complications become established, reversing them is hard, but treatment is available for them early in their course, so watch for them five years after your initial diagnosis of diabetes. See Dr. Rubin's book *Diabetes For Dummies,* 4th Edition (Wiley), for information on screening for these complications.

The long-term complications are divided into two groups: *microvascular,* which are due at least in part to small blood vessel damage, and *macrovascular,* associated with damage to large blood vessels.

Microvascular complications include the following:

- ✔ **Diabetic retinopathy:** Eye damage that leads to blindness if untreated.

- ✔ **Diabetic nephropathy:** Kidney damage that can lead to kidney failure.

- ✔ **Diabetic neuropathy:** Nerve damage that results in many clinical symptoms, the most common of which are tingling and numbness in the feet. Lack of sensation in the feet can result in severe injury without awareness unless you carefully look at your feet regularly. Such injury can result in infection and even amputation.

Macrovascular complications also occur in prediabetes and consist of the following:

- ✔ **Arteriosclerotic heart disease:** Blockage of the blood vessels of the heart. This is the most common cause of death in diabetes due to a heart attack.

- ✔ **Arteriosclerotic cerebrovascular disease:** Blockage of blood vessels to the brain, resulting in a stroke.

- ✔ **Arteriosclerotic peripheral vascular disease involving the blood vessels of the legs:** These vessels can become clogged and result in amputation of the feet or legs.

There is a lot of good news with respect to these complications. According to a study published in the *New England Journal of Medicine* in April 2014, the rates of lower-extremity amputation, end-stage kidney disease, heart attack, stroke, and death from hyperglycemic crisis (ketoacidosis and hyperosmolar syndrome) have all declined between 1990 and 2010. The largest decline was a reduction of 64 percent in heart attacks. The smallest decline was in end-stage renal disease at 28 percent. Furthermore, 30-year follow-up of the people involved in the Diabetes Control and Complications Trial shows that those whose A1C was kept as close to normal as possible during the six and a half years of the trial continued to have a significant reduction in eye and kidney disease of 50 percent, in nerve disease of 30 percent, and in heart attacks of 42 percent. This protection continued despite the fact that the A1C of the intensively treated group converged with that of the conventionally treated group when the study ended.

Recognizing you can manage diabetes

Treatment of diabetes involves three essential elements:

- ✔ **Diet:** If you follow the recommendations in this book, you can lower your average blood glucose by as much as 30 to 50 mg/dl. Doing so can reduce the complication rate by as much as 33 percent.

> ✔ **Exercise:** We touch on exercise in Chapter 3 and Dr. Rubin covers it more extensively in *Diabetes For Dummies,* 4th Edition (Wiley).
>
> ✔ **Medication:** Diabetes medications abound — there are far too many to discuss here, but you can find out about them in *Diabetes For Dummies,* 4th Edition.

Controlling Calories

Just as the three most important factors in the value of a house are location, location, location, the three most important factors in diet for people with diabetes are moderation, moderation, moderation. If you're overweight or obese, which is true of most people with type 2 diabetes and a lot of people with type 1 diabetes who are on intensive insulin treatment (four shots of insulin daily), weight loss will make a huge difference in your blood glucose levels. If you maintain the weight loss, you'll avoid the complications of diabetes discussed earlier in this chapter.

To successfully lose weight, you need to control your total calories. You must burn up the same amount of calories you take in by mouth, or you will gain weight. To lose weight, you need to burn up more calories than you eat. Sounds simple, eh! And it doesn't matter where the calories come from. Studies that compare diets low in fats, proteins, or carbohydrates result in the same weight loss after a year.

As you reduce your portions, reduce your intake of added sugars, fats, and alcohol. These items contain no nutrients such as vitamins and minerals and are simply sources of empty calories.

If you are predisposed to have diabetes because, for example, your parents both had diabetes, you can prevent it by maintaining a healthy weight. If you already have diabetes, you can minimize its impact by losing weight and keeping it off.

Do you need a highly complicated formula to figure out how to moderate your food intake? No! It's as simple as looking at the portions you currently eat and cutting them in half. At home, where you control the amount of food on your plate, you can start with a small portion, so you may not need to reduce it by half. However, in restaurants, where more and more people are eating their meals, especially the fast-food restaurants, discussed extensively in Chapters 17 and 18, the rule of eating half may not be strong enough. There you may need to eat only a third of the portion. You may need to apply the same portion control when you eat at someone else's home.

Use these tips to help you visualize portion sizes:

✔ An ounce of meat is the size of a pack of matches.

✔ Three ounces of meat is the size of a deck of cards.

✔ A medium fruit is the size of a tennis ball.

✔ A medium potato is the size of a computer mouse.

✔ A medium bagel is the size of a hockey puck.

✔ An ounce of cheese is the size of a domino.

✔ A cup of fruit is the size of a baseball.

✔ A cup of broccoli is the size of a light bulb.

You don't need to take in many extra calories over time to gain weight. Just 100 extra kilocalories (see the "Kilocalories versus calories" sidebar for an explanation of kilocalories) on a daily basis results in a weight gain of 12 pounds in a year. An extra glass of wine is that many kilocalories. On the other hand, if you reduce your daily intake by 100 kilocalories, you can lose those 12 pounds over a year.

Look at a few examples of the portion sizes provided today compared to 20 years ago. Table 1-1 shows the kilocalories in the portions of 20 years ago and today and how much exercise you have to do to burn up the extra kilocalories so you don't gain weight.

Table 1-1	Consequences of Today's Larger Portions		
Food	*Kilocalories 20 years ago*	*Kilocalories today*	*Exercise to burn the difference*
Bagel	140	350	50 minutes raking leaves
Cheeseburger	333	590	90 minutes lifting weights
French fries	210	610	80 minutes walking
Turkey sandwich	320	820	85 minutes biking
Coffee	45	350	70 minutes walking
Chicken Caesar salad	390	790	80 minutes walking
Popcorn	270	630	75 minutes of water aerobics
Chocolate chip cookie	55	275	75 minutes washing the car

Kilocalories versus calories

We use the term *kilocalories* (or *kcalories*) rather than calories because experts in health and medicine measure energy in a diet plan or in food in kilocalories (a kilocalorie is 1,000 times greater than a calorie). Unfortunately, the term *calories* has been established on food labels and in diets,

and health officials don't want to confuse the public by attempting to correct this error.

Calorie counts in the text of this book and in the nutritional analyses of the recipes are given in kilocalories.

Moving and Resting

Exercise is just as important as diet in controlling your blood glucose. A group of people who were expected to develop diabetes because their parents both had diabetes was asked to walk 30 minutes a day. Eighty percent of those who did walk did not develop the disease. These people didn't necessarily lose weight, but they did exercise.

Too many people complain that they just can't find the time to exercise. But a recent study showed that just 7½ minutes of highly intense exercise a week had a profound effect on the blood glucose. So this excuse isn't acceptable, especially when you realize how much difference exercise can make in your life and your diabetes. Here are some ways that different amounts of exercise can help you:

- ✔ Thirty minutes of exercise a day will get you in excellent physical shape and reduce your blood glucose substantially.
- ✔ Sixty minutes of exercise a day will help you to maintain weight loss and get you in even better physical shape.
- ✔ Ninety minutes of exercise a day will cause you to lose weight.

An exercise partner helps ensure that you get out and do your thing. We find it extremely helpful to have someone waiting for us so that we can exercise together.

Here are some more facts about exercise to keep in mind:

- ✔ You don't have to get in all your minutes of exercise in one session. Two 30-minute workouts are just as good as and possibly better than one 60-minute workout.

✔ Although walking is excellent exercise, especially for the older population, the benefits of more vigorous exercise and for a longer time are greater still.

✔ Everything counts when it comes to exercise. Your decision to take the stairs instead of the elevator may not seem like much, but if you do so day after day, it makes a profound difference. Another suggestion that may help over time is to park your car farther from your office or bike to the office.

✔ A pedometer (a small gadget worn on your belt that counts your steps) may help you to achieve your exercise goals. The objective is to get up to 10,000 steps a day by increasing your step count every week.

You also want to do something to strengthen your muscles. Larger muscles take in more glucose, providing another way of keeping it under control. You'll be surprised by how much your stamina will increase and how much your blood glucose will fall. Resistance training (weight lifting) may be just as important as aerobic exercise in improving diabetic control. In the Nurses' Health Study, for example, resistance training resulted in a substantial reduction in the occurrence of diabetes.

Place a daily limit on activities that are completely sedentary, such as watching television or surfing the web. Use the time you might have once spent on these activities to exercise. This advice is especially helpful for overweight children who should be limited to two hours a day.

Keeping up to speed on treatment developments

By the time you read this book, several months will have passed since we wrote these words. Several important discoveries about diabetes or related medical information may have occurred that you need to know about. How can you keep up with the latest and greatest treatments?

✔ Take a course with a certified diabetes educator (CDE). Here you learn how to manage your diabetes right now and find out about what's coming up.

✔ Go to the web and do a search for diabetes. If you want to be sure that the sites you come

up with are both accurate and helpful, go to Dr. Rubin's website, www.drrubin.com, where you'll find a page on Useful Diabetes Related websites. He has checked all of them out for you, so you know you can rely on them.

✔ Come to your doctor prepared to ask questions. If you don't get a satisfactory answer, see a specialist.

✔ Take another certified course after several years. You'll be amazed at the changes.

You want to be active, but don't do it at the cost of getting plenty of rest each day. People who sleep eight hours a night tend to be less hungry and leaner than people who sleep less.

Of course, it is possible to overdo it. One French diplomat found the phenomenal energy of President Theodore Roosevelt too much for him. After two sets of tennis at the White House, Roosevelt invited him to go jogging. Then they had a workout with a medicine ball. "What would you like to do now?" the President asked his guest when his enthusiasm for the exercise seemed to be flagging. "If it's all the same to you," gasped the exhausted Frenchman, "lie down and die."

Knowing the New Blood Pressure Limits

Keeping your blood pressure in check is particularly important in preventing the macrovascular complications of diabetes. But elevated blood pressure also plays a role in bringing on eye disease, kidney disease, and neuropathy. You should have your blood pressure tested every time you see your doctor.

Studies have shown that previous blood pressure goals were not significantly more beneficial and did raise the risk of low blood pressure, fainting, and dizziness. The new goal is to keep your blood pressure under 140/80. (See Dr. Rubin's book *High Blood Pressure For Dummies,* 2nd Edition, published by Wiley, for a complete explanation of the meaning of these numbers.) You may want to get your own blood pressure monitor so that you can check it at home yourself.

The statistics about diabetes and high blood pressure are daunting. Seventy-one percent of diabetics have high blood pressure, but almost a third are unaware of it. Almost half of them weren't being treated for high blood pressure. Among the treated patients, less than half were treated in a way that reduced their pressure to lower than 130/80.

You can do plenty of things to lower your blood pressure, including losing weight, avoiding salt, eating more fruits and vegetables, and, of course, exercising. But if all else fails, your doctor may prescribe medication. Many blood pressure medicines are available, and one or two will be exactly right for you. See *High Blood Pressure For Dummies,* 2nd Edition, for an extensive discussion of the large number of blood pressure medications.

One class of drugs in particular is very useful for people with diabetes with high blood pressure: angiotensin converting enzyme inhibitors (ACE inhibitors), which are especially protective of your kidneys. If kidney damage is detected early, ACE inhibitors can reverse the damage. Some experts believe that all diabetics should take ACE inhibitors. We believe that if there's no evidence of kidney damage and the diabetes is well controlled, this isn't necessary.

Accounting for the Rest of Your Lifestyle

Diabetes is just one part of your life. It can affect the rest of your lifestyle, however, and your lifestyle certainly affects your diabetes. In this section, we take up some of these other parts of your lifestyle, all of which you can alter to the benefit of your health and your diabetes.

A good place to start is with alcohol. A glass of wine is a pleasant addition to dinner, and studies show that alcohol in moderation can lower the risk of a heart attack. For a diabetic, it is especially important that food accompany the wine because alcohol reduces the blood glucose; a complication called hypoglycemia may occur (see the section "Short-term complications," earlier in this chapter).

Never drink alcohol without food, especially when you're taking glucose-lowering medication.

The following people should not drink alcohol at all:

✔ Pregnant women

✔ Women who are breastfeeding

✔ Children and adolescents

✔ People who take medications that interact with alcohol

✔ People with medical conditions that are worsened by alcohol, such as liver disease and certain diseases of the pancreas

The amount of wine that is safe on a daily basis is a maximum of two 4-ounce glasses for a man or one 4-ounce glass for a woman. Men metabolize alcohol more rapidly than women, so they can drink more. But you should drink no more than a maximum of five days out of seven.

In terms of alcohol content, 1½ ounces of hard liquor, such as gin, rum, vodka, or whisky, or 12 ounces of light beer are the equivalent of a 4-ounce glass of wine.

Alcohol adds calories without any nutrition. Alcohol has no vitamins or minerals, but you do have to account for the calories in your diet. If you stop drinking alcohol, you may lose a significant amount of weight. For example, a person who has been drinking three drinks a night and stops will lose 26 pounds in a year.

Alcohol can cause cirrhosis of the liver and raises blood pressure. It also worsens diabetic neuropathy. Do you need any more reasons not to drink alcohol?

In addition to drinking alcohol in moderation, here are major ways you can improve the rest of your lifestyle:

✔ Avoid tobacco in any form. It is the number-one killer.

✔ Avoid illicit drugs.

✔ Drive safely.

✔ Benefit from relationships.

✔ Maintain your sense of humor.

Try making changes one at a time, and when you think you have that one under control, move on to the next.

Chapter 2

How What You Eat Affects Your Diabetes

*O*besity is getting bigger. As defined by a body mass index (BMI) of 30 or greater, the percent of Americans who were obese went from 25.6 in 2007 to 35.1 in 2012. During the same period, the prevalence of people with a diagnosis of diabetes went from 23.6 million in 2007 to 26 million in 2012. Sixty-nine percent of the U.S. population is considered overweight (BMI between 25 and 29.9) or obese (BMI of 30 or higher).

The United States must reverse this trend. Otherwise, millions of people will become blind, develop kidney failure, and require amputations. In addition, millions of people will become heart attack victims, many of whom will not survive their first heart attack.

Diet can lower the hemoglobin A1c, a measure of the average glucose in the blood for the last 90 days, by 1 percent or more. For every 1 percent reduction in hemoglobin A1c, there is a 33 percent reduction in complications of diabetes. See *Diabetes For Dummies,* 4th Edition (Wiley), for more information on hemoglobin A1c.

This chapter tells you how much to eat, what to eat, and when to eat. Because most people with diabetes are overweight, we provide advice so that eating healthy becomes a way of life for you. And don't forget the important value of exercise, particularly "skipping" soda, "skipping" fatty foods, and "skipping" desserts.

The first thing you need to know when you plan your diet is how much you should be eating. To find out how many *kilocalories* (commonly called *calories*) you need, you have to do a little math. Chapter 3 shows you how to determine your ideal weight and the number of kilocalories you need, depending on your lifestyle and weight goals.

After you know your total calorie intake objective, break it down into the three sources of energy: carbohydrates, protein, and fat.

Switching to a Mediterranean Diet

In the last edition of this book, we emphasized vegetarian eating as an excellent way to prevent diabetes or to manage it if it occurs. Although a vegetarian diet remains an excellent diet for diabetes, most people prefer to have some animal protein in their diets — for taste, variety, and convenience. The Mediterranean diet fulfills all these criteria and more.

The first big study confirming the benefits of the Mediterranean diet was published in the *Archives of Internal Medicine* in December 2007. It showed a significant reduction in deaths from all causes. More recently, in a study published in the *Annals of Internal Medicine* in January 2014, patients who followed a Mediterranean diet supplemented with extra-virgin olive oil had a significant reduction in the onset of diabetes compared to a control group who were just given advice on a lowfat diet. Another study, published in *Diabetologica* in December 2013, confirmed the advantages of the Mediterranean diet. These are just a few of the many studies pointing to the effectiveness of the Mediterranean diet in preventing or managing diabetes.

What are the major features of the Mediterranean diet? The diet emphasizes the following:

- Plant-based foods such as fruits and vegetables, whole grains, legumes, and nuts
- Olive oil in place of butter or margarine
- Herbs and spices to flavor foods instead of salt
- Red meat no more often than twice a month
- Fish and/or poultry twice a week
- Alcohol in moderation (5 ounces of red wine daily for all women and men over 65 years and 10 ounces for men younger than 65)

Note: People with a family history of alcohol abuse or heart or liver disease should not drink any alcohol.

How can you get started without moving to Greece? Here are some suggestions:

✔ Make sure that most of your meal and snacks are made up of fruits and vegetables, preferably unprocessed and whole. If you eat bread or cereal, make sure it's whole grain. The same is true for rice and pasta.

✔ Skip butter and use olive oil on bread or pasta instead. *Tahini* (blended sesame seeds) is another great alternative to butter.

✔ Eat a handful of almonds, cashews, pistachios, and walnuts for a delicious snack.

✔ Add herbs and spices to flavor your foods.

✔ Grill or bake fish instead of frying or breading it. Especially good for you are tuna, salmon, trout, mackerel, and herring, fresh or in cans.

✔ If you eat dairy, opt for lowfat options like skim milk, fat-free yogurt, and lowfat cheese.

The food that you find in Italian chain restaurants across the United States is not Mediterranean food. They use a lot of butter, full-fat cheese, cream sauce, meat, and white-flour pasta among other non-Mediterranean foods. So, don't think you're eating Mediterranean just because the restaurant serves pasta.

Adding Up Carbohydrates — Precursors of Glucose

When you eat a meal, the immediate source of glucose in your blood comes from the carbohydrates in that meal. One group of carbohydrates is the starches, such as cereals, grains, pastas, breads, crackers, starchy vegetables, beans, peas, and lentils. Fruits make up a second major source of carbohydrate. Milk and milk products contain not only carbohydrate but also protein and a variable amount of fat, depending on whether the milk is whole, lowfat, or fat-free. Other sources of carbohydrate include cakes, cookies, candies, sweetened beverages, and ice cream. These foods also contain a variable amount of fat.

To determine what else is found in food, check a source such as *The Official Pocket Guide to Diabetic Exchanges,* published by the American Diabetes Association and the American Dietetic Association, or *The Diabetes Carbohydrate and Fat Gram Guide,* published by the American Diabetes Association.

Determining the amount of carbohydrate: Does it matter?

For decades, the American Diabetes Association (ADA) has been recommending specific percentages of each macronutrient — carbohydrate, protein, and fat — for people with diabetes. After completely reviewing the evidence, the ADA has concluded in its Clinical Practice Recommendations for 2014,

> . . . there is not an ideal percentage of calories from carbohydrate, protein, and fat for all people with diabetes; therefore, macronutrient distribution should be based on individualized assessment of current eating patterns, preferences, and metabolic goals.

If this feels a little vague to you, and you'd like some more concrete guidelines, here's what a typical day on a Mediterranean diet looks like, along with the breakdown of macronutrients for that day:

- ✔ **Breakfast:** 1 cup nonfat yogurt with ¾ cup berries and 1 slice wholewheat bread with 2 tablespoons hummus
- ✔ **Snack:** 1 apple
- ✔ **Lunch:** 4 ounces salmon with herbs grilled in olive oil with baked kale, ½ cup peas
- ✔ **Snack:** 6 almonds and ¼ cup grapes
- ✔ **Dinner:** 4 ounces white-meat chicken with rosemary, ⅓ cup brown rice and broccoli, 1 slice whole-wheat bread, and a glass of red wine
- ✔ **Snack:** 4 crackers with 4 ounces lowfat cheese

This day of a Mediterranean diet is 45 percent carbohydrate, 25 percent protein, and 30 percent fat.

You don't have to stick to these percentages — this is just one example of a typical day on the Mediterranean diet.

Considering the glycemic index

The various carbohydrate sources differ in the degree to which they raise the blood glucose. This difference is called the *glycemic index* (GI), and it refers to the glucose-raising power of a food compared with white bread.

In general, choose foods with a lower glycemic index in order to keep the rise in blood glucose to a minimum. Predicting the glycemic index of a mixed meal (one that contains an appetizer, a main dish, and a dessert) is nearly impossible, but you can make some simple substitutions to lower the glycemic index of your diet, as shown in Table 2-1. These substitutions are very much in keeping with the Mediterranean diet.

Table 2-1	Simple Diet Substitutions to Lower GI
High GI foods	*Low GI foods*
Whole meal or white bread	Whole-grain bread
Processed breakfast cereal	Unrefined cereals like oats or processed low-GI cereals
Plain cookies and crackers	Cookies made with dried fruits or whole grains like oats
Cakes and muffins	Cakes and muffins made with fruits, oats, and whole grains
Tropical fruits like bananas	Temperate-climate fruits like apples and plums
Potatoes	Whole-wheat pasta or legumes
Rice	Basmati, brown rice, long-grain rice, or other low-GI rice

Many of these lower glycemic index foods contain a lot of fiber. Fiber is a carbohydrate that can't be broken down by digestive enzymes, so it doesn't raise blood glucose and adds no calories. Fiber has been shown to reduce the risk of coronary heart disease and diabetes while it improves bowel function, preventing constipation. For the person who has diabetes already, fiber reduces blood glucose levels. The riper the fruit, the higher the GI.

If a food has a lot of fiber in it (more than 5 grams per serving), you can subtract the grams of fiber from the grams of carbohydrates in that food in determining the calories from carbohydrate.

The best sources of fiber are fruits, whole grains, and vegetables, especially the legumes. Animal food sources don't provide fiber. It is recommended that you consume 25 grams of fiber daily. Table 2-2 shows some sources of larger amounts of fiber.

Table 2-2	Sources of Fiber	
Food, Amount	*Fiber (g)*	*Kcalories*
Navy beans, cooked, ½ cup	9.5	128
Bran cereal, ½ cup	8.8	78
Kidney beans, ½ cup	8.2	109
Split peas, cooked, ½ cup	8.1	116
Lentils, cooked ½ cup	7.8	115
Black beans, cooked, ½ cup	7.5	114
Whole-wheat English muffin	4.4	134
Pear, raw, small	4.3	81
Apple, with skin, 1 medium	3.3	72

Fiber can be present in two forms:

- ✔ **Insoluble:** It doesn't dissolve in water but stays in the intestine as *roughage,* which helps to prevent constipation; for example, fiber found in whole-grain breads and cereals, and the skin of fruits and vegetables.

- ✔ **Soluble:** It dissolves in water and enters the blood, where it helps lower glucose and cholesterol; for example, fiber found in barley, brown rice, and beans, as well as vegetables and fruits.

You can take a spoonful of sugar in your coffee and have a little sugar in your food, but be aware of the number of calories you are adding with no micronutrients (vitamins and minerals present in tiny amounts but essential). See "Monitoring Your Micronutrients," later in this chapter, for more info.

Choosing sugar substitutes

Although people with diabetes are allowed to have some sugar in their diet, sugar is more appropriate for a diabetic who is at normal weight than an obese diabetic. Preventing obesity may be a matter of avoiding as little as 50 extra calories a day. If this can be accomplished by using artificial sweeteners, which provide sweetening power but no calories, so much the better.

There is no good evidence that using sugar substitutes results in significant weight loss.

Some of the recipes in this book call for ¼ cup or more of sugar. These are perfect opportunities to use a sugar substitute and significantly lower the calories from sugar.

Kilocalorie-containing sweeteners

Several sugars besides sucrose (table sugar) are present in food. These sugars have different properties than glucose, are taken up differently from the intestine, and raise the blood level at a slower rate or not at all if they're not ultimately converted into glucose. They sometimes cause diarrhea.

Although these kilocalorie-containing sweeteners are sweeter than sugar and you use them in smaller amounts, they *do* have calories that you must count in your daily intake.

The following sweeteners contain kilocalories but act differently in the body than sucrose:

✔ **Fructose, found in fruits and berries:** Fructose is sweeter than table sugar and is absorbed more slowly than glucose, so it raises the glucose level more slowly. When it enters the bloodstream, it is taken up by the liver, where it is converted to glucose.

✔ **Xylitol, found in strawberries and raspberries:** Xylitol is also sweeter than table sugar and has fewer kilocalories per gram. It is absorbed more slowly than sugar. When used in gum, for example, it reduces the occurrence of dental caries (tooth decay).

✔ **Sorbitol and mannitol, sugar alcohols occurring in plants:** Sorbitol and mannitol are half as sweet as table sugar and have little effect on blood glucose. They change to fructose in the body.

Sweeteners without calories

This group of non-nutritive or artificial sweeteners (with the exception of Stevia, which comes from a plant) is much sweeter than table sugar and contains no calories at all. Much less of these sweeteners will provide the same level of sweetness as a larger amount of sugar. However, the taste of some of them may seem a little "off" compared to sugar or honey. They include the following:

✔ **Saccharin:** This has 300 to 400 times the sweetening power of sugar, and it is heat stable so it can be used in baking and cooking. Brand names for saccharin are Sucaryl, SugarTwin, and Sweet'N Low.

✔ **Aspartame:** This is more expensive than saccharin, but people often prefer its taste. It is 150 to 200 times as sweet as sugar. Equal and Sweet Mate are two of the brands. It loses its sweetening power when heated, so it can't be used if food has to be cooked for longer than 20 minutes.

✔ **Acesulfame-K:** This is 200 times sweeter than sugar and is heat stable, so it is used in baking and cooking.

✔ **Stevia:** This is 250 to 300 times sweeter than sugar. It was approved by the FDA in 2008 and marketed as Rebiana in Coca-Cola.

✔ **Sucralose:** This sweetener, which is made from sugar, is 600 times sweeter than its parent, sucrose. The brand name is Splenda. It remains stable when heated and has become a favorite sweetener in the food industry. Because foods don't bake the same when made with Splenda, a combination of Splenda and sugar called "Pure Magic" is sold to reduce calories while providing the baking characteristics of sugar.

Appendix C shows the amount of these various sweeteners that will give the sweetening power of a measured amount of sucrose (table sugar). Feel free to substitute calorie-free sweeteners whenever sugar is called for. The calories you save could make a big difference in your diabetes.

Contrary to opinions that you may hear or read, there is no scientific evidence that these sweeteners are associated with a higher incidence of cancer.

Eating Enough Protein (Preferably Not from Red Meat)

Protein comes from meat, fish, poultry, milk, and cheese. It can also be found in beans, peas, and lentils, which we mention in the carbohydrate discussion in the preceding section. Meat sources of protein can be low or very high in fat, depending on the source. Because people with diabetes should be trying to keep the fat content of their diets fairly low, lowfat sources of protein, such as skinless white meat chicken or turkey, flounder or halibut, and fat-free cheese are preferred. Beans, peas, and lentils, which can be very good sources of protein, don't contain fat but do contain carbohydrate.

Protein doesn't cause an immediate rise in blood glucose, but it can raise glucose levels several hours later, after your liver processes the protein and converts some of it into glucose. Therefore, protein isn't a good choice if you want to treat low blood glucose, but a snack containing protein at bedtime may help prevent low blood glucose during the night.

Focusing on Fat and Using Statins

Fat comes in many different forms. The one everyone talks about is cholesterol, the type found in the yolk of an egg. However, most of the fat that people eat comes in a chemical form known as triglyceride. This term refers to the chemistry of the fat, and we don't have to get into the details of it for you to understand how to handle fat in your diet. In the following sections, we start with a discussion of cholesterol and then turn to other forms of fat.

Zeroing in on cholesterol

These days, just about everyone knows his or her cholesterol level. You usually find out your total cholesterol level, a combination of so-called good cholesterol and bad cholesterol. If your total is high, much of that cholesterol may be the good kind — *HDL (high-density lipoprotein)* cholesterol. If you're interested in knowing the balance between good and bad cholesterol in your body, talk with your medical practitioner, who may recommend a *lipid panel*, a blood test that delivers more details.

The Framingham Study, an ongoing study of the health of the citizens of Framingham, Massachusetts, has shown that the total cholesterol amount divided by the good cholesterol figure gives a number that is a reasonable measure of the risk of a heart attack. People who had results that were less than 4.5 were at lower risk of heart attacks, while those with results of more that 4.5 were at higher risk. The risk increases as the number rises.

More recently, another component of the total cholesterol in your blood, the so-called bad cholesterol or *LDL-C (low-density lipoprotein cholesterol)* has been found to have a very important role in causing heart attacks. For people at high risk of a heart attack, the recommended level for LDL used to be less than 100 mg/dl but has recently been lowered to less than 70 mg/dl.

Most foods don't contain much cholesterol — with the exception of eggs. The daily recommendation for cholesterol is less than 300 milligrams, and one egg almost reaches that level. Some doctors say that eating an egg two or three times a week won't hurt you, but this isn't true if you have diabetes. Avoid eggs and foods such as organ meats that are high in cholesterol, or use egg substitutes instead.

When total and bad cholesterol levels are too high, drugs called *statins* are usually given, especially to people with diabetes. Recently, new guidelines have been published by the American Heart Association for the use of statins. The guidelines depend on a ten-year risk calculator that can be found at: `http://my.americanheart.org/professional/ StatementsGuidelines/Prevention-Guidelines_UCM_457698_ SubHomePage.jsp`. The following four groups are recommended to have statin therapy:

✔ People without cardiovascular disease who are 40 to 75 years old and have a 7.5 percent or higher risk for a stroke or heart attack in the next ten years

✔ People with a history of a cardiovascular event such as a stroke or heart attack

✔ People 21 and older who have a very high level of bad cholesterol (190 mg/dl or higher)

✔ People with Type 1 or Type 2 diabetes who are 40 to 75 years old

The last criteria means that just about every person with diabetes should eventually be on statins.

The guidelines also state that patients on statins no longer need to get LDL cholesterol down to a specific target number. This means that when you're on statins, you rarely, if ever, need to be retested. And the guidelines recommend that it isn't necessary to add other cholesterol-lowering drugs because they haven't been shown to reduce heart attack or stroke risk.

Taking a look at other types of fat

Although cholesterol gets all the press, most of the fat you eat is in the form of triglyceride, the fat you see on fatty meats, contained in whole-fat dairy products, and in many processed foods. There are several forms of triglyceride:

✔ **Saturated fat** is the kind of fat that comes from animal sources like that big piece of rib-eye steak you ate the other night. Butter, bacon, cream, and cream cheese are other examples. Saturated fat increases your bad cholesterol levels and should be avoided.

✔ **Trans fats** were invented by food manufacturers to replace butter, which is more expensive. Unfortunately trans fats, which are currently listed as partially hydrogenated oil on food labels, may be worse than saturated fat in causing coronary heart disease. They're found in margarine, cake mixes, dried soup mixes, many fast foods, and many frozen foods, doughnuts, cookies, potato chips, breakfast cereals, candies, and whipped toppings. Food manufacturers have been removing trans fats from numerous foods, but you still may find then in fried foods in restaurants. Keep them out of your diet by reading food labels, which must list them.

✔ **Unsaturated fats** come from vegetable sources such as olive oil and canola oil. There are two forms of unsaturated fats:

  • **Monounsaturated fats,** which don't raise cholesterol in the blood. Olive oil, canola oil, and avocado are some examples. The oil in nuts is also monounsaturated.

  • **Polyunsaturated fats,** which don't raise cholesterol but can lower good or HDL cholesterol. Corn oil, mayonnaise, and some margarines have this form of fat.

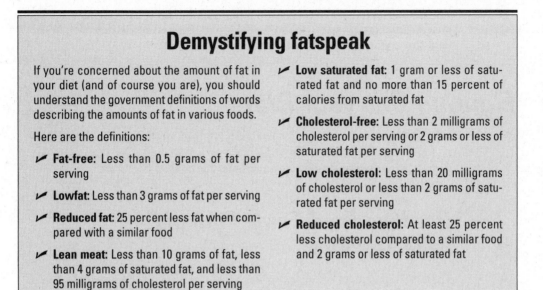

Demystifying fatspeak

If you're concerned about the amount of fat in your diet (and of course you are), you should understand the government definitions of words describing the amounts of fat in various foods.

Here are the definitions:

✔ **Fat-free:** Less than 0.5 grams of fat per serving

✔ **Lowfat:** Less than 3 grams of fat per serving

✔ **Reduced fat:** 25 percent less fat when compared with a similar food

✔ **Lean meat:** Less than 10 grams of fat, less than 4 grams of saturated fat, and less than 95 milligrams of cholesterol per serving

✔ **Low saturated fat:** 1 gram or less of saturated fat and no more than 15 percent of calories from saturated fat

✔ **Cholesterol-free:** Less than 2 milligrams of cholesterol per serving or 2 grams or less of saturated fat per serving

✔ **Low cholesterol:** Less than 20 milligrams of cholesterol or less than 2 grams of saturated fat per serving

✔ **Reduced cholesterol:** At least 25 percent less cholesterol compared to a similar food and 2 grams or less of saturated fat

Curbing your fat intake

Fat has concentrated calories, so don't eat too much fat in your diet. However, monounsaturated fats seem to protect against heart disease. The increased intake of olive oil by people living around the Mediterranean Sea may be the reason for their lower incidence of heart disease.

Although vegetable sources of fat are generally better than animal sources, the exceptions are palm oil and coconut oil, which are highly saturated fats.

Here's our bottom-line recommendation: No more than 30 percent of your kilocalories should come from fat, and of that, no more than a third should come from saturated fats. For a person eating 1,500 kilocalories a day, this recommendation would mean 450 kilocalories from fat, and 150 of those kilocalories from saturated fat.

Use vegetable oils, preferably canola oil and olive oil, as your primary sources of fat, because these lower cholesterol.

Choose fish or poultry as your source of protein in order to avoid consuming too much fat along with your protein. If you remove the skin from chicken, you'll get little fat. Fish actually has certain fatty acids that lower cholesterol.

There's a little danger in eating too much salmon, however. One man ate so many salmon croquettes, salmon steaks, and salmon salads that he had to fight the urge to go north and spawn.

Figuring Out Your Diet

After you know how much to eat of each energy source (carbohydrate, fat, and protein), how do you translate this into actual foods? You can use two basic approaches and a new, even simpler technique.

Goodbye Food Guide Pyramid, hello MyPlate

The U.S. Department of Agriculture (USDA) has attempted to simplify people's lives by developing MyPlate in place of the complicated Food Guide Pyramid. Visualize a dinner plate and follow these recommendations:

- ✔ Fill half your plate with fruits and vegetables.
- ✔ Fill one-quarter of your plate with grains and make at least half of those grains whole grains (brown not white rice, whole-wheat bread not white bread).
- ✔ Fill the other one-quarter of your plate with protein daily.
- ✔ At each meal, consume 1 cup of fat-free or lowfat dairy daily. (This is alongside the plate.)
- ✔ Substitute solid fats like butter with oils like olive oil, and eat 6 to 7 teaspoons daily.

The major differences between the USDA MyPlate and a Mediterranean MyPlate are that all the grains for the Mediterranean diet would be whole grains, and red meat would be limited to twice a month.

Working with diabetic exchanges

Diabetic exchanges were first developed by the American Diabetes Association and the U.S. Public Health Service in the 1950s. They were revised in 1976, 1986, and 1995, but dietitians, in general, ignore it in advising patients with diabetes. We believe it is time to drop it from the teaching of good food practices in diabetes. If you have a previous version of this book, please cross it out! Carbohydrate counting, in the next section, is a much simpler and more useful approach.

Counting carbohydrates

People with type 1 diabetes and those with type 2 diabetes who take insulin may find the technique of counting carbohydrates to be the easiest for them. You still need to know how much carbohydrate you should eat in a given day. You divide the total into the meals and snacks that you eat and then, with the help of your doctor or certified diabetes educator, you determine your short-acting insulin needs based upon that amount of carbohydrates and the blood glucose that you measure before that meal.

For example, suppose that a person with diabetes is about to have a break-fast containing 60 grams of carbohydrate. He has found that each unit of lispro insulin controls about 20 grams of carbohydrate intake in his body. Figuring the proper amount of short-acting insulin can be accomplished by a process of trial and error: knowing the amount of carbohydrate intake and determining how many units are needed to keep the blood glucose level about the same after eating the carbohydrate as it was before. (The number of carbohydrate grams that each unit of insulin can control differs for each individual, and another person might control only 15 grams per unit.)

In this example, the person's measured blood glucose is 150 mg/dl (milli-grams per deciliter). This result is about 50 mg/dl higher than he wants it to be. He knows that he can lower his blood glucose by 50 mg/dl for every unit of insulin he takes. Therefore, he needs 3 units of lispro for the carbohydrate intake and 1 unit for the elevated blood glucose for a total of 4 units. For more information on lispro, other types of insulin, and figuring out insulin sensitivity, see Dr. Rubin's book *Diabetes For Dummies,* 4th Edition (Wiley).

He has a morning that is more active than he expected. When lunchtime comes, his blood glucose is down to 60 mg/dl. He's about to eat a lunch con-taining 75 grams of carbohydrate. He takes 4 units of lispro for the food but reduces it by 1 unit to a total of 3 units because his blood glucose is low.

At dinner, he is eating 45 grams of carbohydrate. His blood glucose is 115 mg/dl. He takes 2 units of lispro for the food intake and needs no change for the blood glucose, so he takes only 2 units.

To be a successful carbohydrate counter, you must

✔ Have an accurate knowledge of the grams of carbohydrate in the food you are about to eat and how many units of insulin you need for a given number of grams of carbohydrate.

✔ Measure your blood glucose and know how your body responds to each unit of insulin.

You can make this calculation a little easier by using *constant carbohydrates,* which means that you try to choose carbohydrates so that you are eating about the same amount at every meal and snack. This approach makes determining proper amounts of insulin less tricky; just add or subtract units based upon your blood glucose level before that meal. A few sessions with your physician or a certified diabetes educator can help you feel more comfortable about counting carbohydrates.

Using a simple calculation

For patients with type 1 diabetes and those with type 2 diabetes who take a shot of rapid-acting insulin before meals and a shot of long-acting insulin once a day, this may be the easiest way to go. And it is just as effective as carbohydrate counting in lowering the hemoglobin A1c.

The method is based on a study published in *Diabetes Care* in July 2008. The authors compared their method with a group that did traditional carbohydrate counting and found no difference. Both techniques lowered the hemoglobin A1c into the normal range.

The targets were a fasting blood glucose of less than 95 mg/dl, blood glucose before lunch and dinner of less than 100 mg/dl, and bedtime glucose of less than 130 mg/dl.

The initial dose of the long-acting insulin (in this case, insulin glargine) was determined by adding all the insulin taken in a day before the study began. The dose was then started at 50 percent of the previous total daily insulin. The dose was adjusted by taking the mean of the previous three-day fasting glucose levels. The adjustment was then made as follows:

If the mean of the last three-day fasting glucose was

- ✔ **Greater than 180 mg/dl:** Increase 8 units
- ✔ **140 to 180 mg/dl:** Increase 6 units
- ✔ **120 to 139 mg/dl:** Increase 4 units
- ✔ **95 to 119 mg/dl:** Increase 2 units
- ✔ **70 to 94 mg/dl:** No change
- ✔ **Less than 70 mg/dl:** Decrease by the same units as the previous increase or up to 10 percent of the previous dose

The dose of the rapid-acting insulin before meals (in this case, insulin glulisine) at first totaled the other 50 percent of the pre-study daily insulin. It was divided into 50 percent for the meal with the most carbohydrate, 33 percent for the middle meal, and 17 percent for the meal with the least carbohydrate. Table 2-3 shows the adjustments made to the rapid-acting insulin based on the pattern of the pre-lunch, pre-dinner, and bedtime glucose patterns of the previous week.

Table 2-3	Adjustment of Rapid-Acting Insulin	
Mealtime and bedtime dose	*Pattern of mealtime blood glucose below target*	*Pattern of mealtime blood glucose above target*
Less than or equal to 10 units	Decrease by 1 unit	Increase by 1 unit
11 to 19 units	Decrease by 2 units	Increase by 2 units
20 units or greater	Decrease by 3 units	Increase by 3 units

Try this system for yourself. It's easy and it works.

Monitoring Your Micronutrients

Food contains a lot more than just carbohydrate, protein, and fat. Most of the other components are *micronutrients* (present in tiny or micro quantities), which are essential for maintaining the health of human beings. Examples of micronutrients include vitamins (such as vitamin C and vitamin K) and minerals (such as calcium, magnesium, and iron). Most micronutrients are needed in such small amounts that it's extremely unlikely that you would ever suffer a deficiency of them. A person who eats a balanced diet by using the pyramid technique or the exchange technique doesn't have to worry about getting sufficient quantities of micronutrients — with a few exceptions, which follow:

✔ Adults need to be sure to take in at least 1,000 milligrams of calcium each day. If you're a young person still growing, pregnant, or elderly, you need 1,500 milligrams daily. The best food sources of calcium are plain nonfat yogurt, fat-free or lowfat milk, fortified ready-to-eat cereals, and calcium-fortified soy beverages.

✔ Some menstruating women lose more iron than their bodies can spare and need to take iron supplements. The best sources of iron are iron-rich plant foods like spinach and lowfat meats.

✔ You probably take in 20 to 40 times more salt (sodium) than you need and are better off leaving added salt out of your diet.

✔ You should increase your uptake of potassium to help lower blood pressure. The best sources are leafy green vegetables, fruit from vines, and root vegetables. For more information on micronutrients, check out *Diabetes For Dummies,* 4th Edition.

Coffee and the diabetic

A word or two should definitely be said about consuming coffee and its effect on diabetes. Many studies, the most recent of which is a study in *Diabetes Care* in February 2014, have shown that there is an inverse relationship between consumption of both caffeinated and decaffeinated coffee and the risk of type 2 diabetes. The more coffee consumed, the lower the risk of diabetes. On the other hand, there is some evidence that if you have diabetes, caffeine may raise the blood glucose. The explanation for this paradox is not clear. At present it is up to you.

Recognizing the Importance of Timing of Food and Medication

If you take insulin, the peak of your insulin activity should correspond with the greatest availability of glucose in your blood. To accomplish this, you need to know the time when your insulin is most active, how long it lasts, and when it is no longer active.

- ✔ *Regular insulin,* which has been around for decades, takes 30 minutes to start to lower the glucose level, peaks at three hours, and is gone by six to eight hours. This insulin is used before meals to keep glucose low until the next meal. The problem with regular insulin has always been that you have to take it 30 minutes before you eat or run the risk of becoming hypoglycemic at first, and hyperglycemic later when the insulin is no longer around but your food is providing glucose.

- ✔ *Rapid-acting lispro insulin* and *insulin glulisine* are the newest preparations and the shortest acting. They begin to lower the glucose level within five minutes after administration, peak at about one hour, and are no longer active by about three hours. These insulins are a great advance because they free the person with diabetes to take a shot only when he or she eats. Because their activity begins and ends so quickly, they don't cause hypoglycemia as often as the older preparation.

Given a choice, because of its rapid onset and fall-off in activity, we recommend either lispro or glulisine as the short-acting insulins of choice for people with type 1 diabetes and those with type 2 diabetes who take insulin.

If you're going out to eat, you rarely know when the food will be served. Using rapid-acting insulins, you can measure your blood glucose when the food arrives and take an immediate shot. These preparations really free you to take insulin when you need it. They add a level of flexibility to your schedule that didn't exist before.

If you take regular insulin, keep to a more regular schedule of eating. In addition to short-acting insulin, if you have type 1 diabetes, or in some instances type 2 diabetes, you need to take a longer-acting preparation. The reason is to ensure that some insulin is always circulating to keep your body's metabolism running smoothly. Insulin glargine and insulin detemir are preparations that have no peak of activity but are available for 24 hours. You take one shot daily at bedtime, and they cover your needs for insulin except when large amounts of glucose enter your blood after meals. That is what rapid-acting insulins are for.

Each person responds in his or her own way to different preparations of insulin. You need to test your blood glucose to determine your individual response.

An additional factor affecting the onset of insulin is the location of the injection. Because your abdominal muscles are usually at rest, injection of insulin into the abdomen results in more consistent blood glucose levels. If you use the arms or legs, the insulin will be taken up faster or slower, depending on whether you exercise or not. Be sure to rotate sites.

The depth of the injection also affects the onset of activity of the insulin. A deeper injection results in a faster onset of action. If you use the same length needle and insert it to its maximum length each time, you'll ensure more uniform activity.

You can see from the discussion in this section that a great deal of variation is possible in the taking of an insulin shot. It's no wonder that people who must inject insulin tend to have many more ups and downs in their blood glucose. But with proper education, these variations can be reduced.

If you take oral medication, in particular the sulfonylurea drugs like micronase and glucotrol, the timing of food in relation to the taking of your medication must also be considered. For a complete explanation of this balance between food and medication, see *Diabetes For Dummies,* 4th Edition.

Chapter 3

Planning Meals for Your Weight Goal

● ●

In This Chapter

▶ Deciding how many calories to eat

▶ Shedding weight quickly at 1,200 kilocalories

▶ Dropping weight more slowly at 1,500 kilocalories

▶ Staying at your current weight with 1,800 kilocalories

▶ Looking at other diets

● ●

*Y*ou can eat wisely, get all the nutrients you need, and continue to eat great food, but you do have to limit your portions. In this chapter, we show you how to plan three different daily levels of kilocalories (the proper term for what most people call calories). You can lose weight rapidly, lose more slowly, or maintain your weight.

We prefer the slower approach to losing weight. With this method, you'll probably feel less hungry, and cutting back a few hundred kilocalories a day doesn't cause a major upheaval in daily life. Also, maintaining a weight loss may be easier if you lose the weight slowly, which means you're probably losing fat mass rather than muscle or water.

Exercise can help speed up weight loss or permit you to eat more and still lose weight. Twenty minutes of walking burns up 100 kilocalories, and 30 minutes of walking burns up 150 kilocalories. Walk for 30 minutes a day, and you lose about ⅓ of a pound per week (7 times 150 equals 1,050 kilocalories divided into 3,500) — without reducing your kilocalories. That activity amounts to an annual weight loss of 17 pounds in a year. Who says you can't lose weight by exercising but not dieting?

Considering the calories you're storing

Patients often worry that they're going to feel hungry if they take in fewer calories than they need. Does a bear feel hungry as it lives off its fat all winter long? No, it sleeps.

One of our favorite tasks is to point out how many calories of energy are stored in the body of an overweight or obese person. Each pound of fat contains 3,500 kilocalories. If you're 25 pounds overweight, you have 87,500 kilocalories (25 times 3,500) of stored energy in your body. We can give you an idea of what you could do with that much energy. You need 100 kilocalories to walk 20 minutes at 4 miles an hour. So a walk of 1⅓ miles (one-third of 4 miles) burns 100 kilocalories. Your stored energy — 87,500 kilocalories — would take you about 1,100 miles (87,500 divided by 100 times 1⅓)!

We certainly don't suggest that you stop eating and fast for any length of time in order to lose weight, but recognize that your stored energy, in the form of fat, will provide all the calories necessary to continue your daily activities without fatigue and often without hunger.

Figuring Out How Many Calories You Need

Before planning a nutritional program, you need to know how much you need to eat on a daily basis to maintain your current weight. Then you can figure how rapidly a deficit of calories will get you to your goal.

Finding your ideal weight range

The ideal weight for your height is a range and not a single weight at each height, but we use numbers that give a weight in the middle of that range. Because people have different amounts of muscle and different size frames, you're considered normal if your weight is plus or minus 10 percent of this number. For example, a person who is calculated to have an ideal weight of 150 pounds is considered normal at a weight of 135 (150 minus 10 percent) to 165 (150 plus 10 percent) pounds.

Because no two people, even twins, are totally alike in all aspects of their lives, we can only approximate your ideal weight and the number of calories you need to maintain that weight. You'll test the correctness of the approximation by adding or subtracting calories. If your daily caloric needs are 2,000 kilocalories and you find yourself putting on weight, try reducing your intake by 100 kilocalories and see whether you maintain your weight on fewer kilocalories.

If you're a male, your approximate ideal weight is 106 pounds for 5 feet of height plus 6 pounds for each inch over 5 feet. If you're a female, your ideal weight is 100 pounds for 5 feet plus 5 pounds for each inch over 5 feet tall. For example, a 5-foot-4-inch male should weigh 130 pounds while the same height female should weigh 120 pounds. Your ideal weight range is then plus or minus 10 percent. The male could weigh 117 to 143 pounds and the female 108 to 132 pounds.

Now you know your ideal weight for your height. What a surprise! Yes, we know. You have big bones, but bear with us. It is amazing how often we have seen big bones melt away as weight is lost.

Determining your caloric needs

After you know about how much you should weigh, figure out how many calories you need to maintain your ideal weight. Start by multiplying your ideal weight by ten. For example, if you're a male, 5 feet, 6 inches tall, your ideal weight is 142 pounds. Your daily kilocalorie allowance is about 1,400. But this number is ideal only if you don't take a breath or have a heartbeat. It is considered your *basal* caloric need. You must increase your calorie intake depending upon the amount of physical activity you do each day. Table 3-1 shows this graduated increase.

Table 3-1	Kilocalories Needed Based on Activity Level	
Level of Activity	*Kilocalories Added*	*5'6" Male*
Sedentary	10% more than basal	1,540 kilocalories
Moderate	20% more than basal	1,680 kilocalories
Very active	40%+ more than basal	1,960+ kilocalories

The "Very active" line displays a plus sign because some people doing hard manual labor need so many extra calories that they should not be held to only 40 percent more than their basal calorie intake. This requirement becomes clear as the person gains or loses weight on his or her food plan.

You gain weight when your daily intake of kilocalories exceeds your daily needs. Each pound of fat has 3,500 kilocalories, so when the excess has reached that number of calories, you are a pound heavier. On the other hand, you lose weight when your daily expenditure of calories exceeds your daily intake. You lose a pound of fat each time you burn up 3,500 kilocalories more than you take in, whether you do it by burning an extra 100 kilocalories per day for 35 days or an extra 500 kilocalories per day for 7 days.

Now you can create a nutritional program and fill in the blanks with carbohydrates, proteins, fats, and real foods.

Losing Weight Rapidly at 1,200 Kilocalories

If you're a moderately active male, 5 feet, 6 inches tall, you need 1,680 or approximately 1,700 kilocalories daily to maintain your weight. (Refer to Table 3-2.) If you eat only 1,200 kilocalories daily, you'll have a daily deficit of approximately 500 kilocalories. By dividing the kilocalories in a pound of fat (3,500) by 500, you can see that you'll lose 1 pound per week (3,500 divided by 500 is 7, so the loss will take 7 days).

In Chapter 2, you find that you want to eat 40 percent of your calories as carbohydrate, 30 percent as protein, and 30 percent as fat. Multiplying 1,200 kilocalories by those percentages, a 1,200 kilocalorie diet would provide 480 kilocalories of carbohydrate, 360 kilocalories of protein, and 360 kilocalories of fat. Because there are 4 kilocalories of energy in each gram of carbohydrate and protein, dividing the kilocalories by 4, you can eat 120 grams of carbohydrate and 90 grams of protein. Because there are 9 kilocalories in each gram of fat, you can eat 40 grams of fat.

You can create your diet using recipes where you know the grams of carbohydrate, such as the ones in this book. Table 3-2 shows you such a diet.

Table 3-2	A 1,200-Kilocalorie Diet			
Meal	*Recipe*	*Carbs (g)*	*Protein (g)*	*Fat (g)*
Breakfast	Whole-Wheat Waffles (Chapter 6)	30	9	1
Lunch	Goat-Cheese-Stuffed Zucchini with Yellow Tomato Sauce (Chapter 11)	17	21	30
Dinner	Horseradish-Crusted Cod with Lentils (Chapter 12)	73	58	9
Total		**120**	**88**	**40**

All we did in making up this diet was to make sure the carbohydrate total came to about 120 grams. It was purely accidental that the grams of protein and fat worked out so well. If they had not, the next day's diet would have been more of what was missing and less of what was present in too large an amount.

You can see how easy it is to create a diet when the grams of protein, fat, and carbohydrate are listed for you as they are in this book. It is very difficult to do the same thing when you go to a restaurant and have no idea of the contents of the food. At the grocery store, the food label gives you the breakdown that you need. That is why it is so important to check the food labels, as explained in Chapter 5, to find out how much carbohydrate, protein, and fat the food actually contains.

The portions on all food labels are based on a 2,000-kilocalorie diet. Not one of the diets in this chapter allows you to eat that many calories. Such a portion may be much too large for a person on a 1,200-kilocalorie diet.

Losing Weight More Slowly at 1,500 Kilocalories

The smaller the deficit of calories between what you need and what you eat, the more slowly you'll lose weight. If your daily needs are 1,700 kilocalories and you eat 1,500, you'll be missing 200 kilocalories each day. Because a pound of fat is 3,500 kilocalories, you'll lose a pound in about 17 days (3,500 divided by 200). You'll lose almost 2 pounds a month, or 24 pounds in a year. You can accomplish this loss by reducing your daily intake by only the equivalent of a piece of bread and two teaspoons of margarine. Put that way, losing the weight doesn't seem difficult at all.

In Table 3-3, we use the recipes in this book to make up a 1,500-kilocalorie diet. In this plan, you're eating 600 kilocalories of carbohydrate or 150 grams, 450 kilocalories of protein or 112 grams, and 450 kilocalories of fat or 50 grams.

Table 3-3	A 1,500-Kilocalorie Diet			
Meal	*Recipe*	*Carbs (g)*	*Protein (g)*	*Fat (g)*
Breakfast	Blueberry and Almond Pancakes (Chapter 6)	38	10	2
Lunch	Indian-Inspired Lamb and Legume Chile (Chapter 8)	23	23	14
Dinner	Paillard of Chicken Breast with Fennel and Parmigiano (Chapter 13)	24	51	33
Total		**85**	**84**	**49**

You notice that this plan is 65 grams low on carbohydrate, 28 grams low on protein, and 1 gram low on fat. This allows you to have some fruit with the meal or snacks in between to make up the difference. An apple, half banana, and 12 cherries will provide 45 grams of carbohydrate because each is 15 grams. A tablespoon of cashews and 6 almonds will provide 10 grams of unsaturated fat. Two ounces of ricotta cheese with 5 grams of fat per ounce will provide 10 grams of fat.

As you create your meals, you'll be amazed at how small the portions really are. Four ounces of lean meat isn't much compared to what most people are used to eating at home or in restaurants. Eating proper portions is very important because it will ultimately make the difference between weight gain and weight maintenance or loss. Portion size may also be the difference between controlling your blood glucose and not controlling it. Check out Chapter 1 for more about portion sizes.

Think of the money you will save if — each time you go to a restaurant — your knowledge of portion sizes allows you to take home half of your meal to eat another day.

Maintaining Your Weight at 1,800 Kilocalories

Suppose that you have finally reached a weight (not necessarily your "ideal" weight that we calculate in the section "Figuring Your Daily Caloric Needs") that allows your blood glucose levels to remain between 80 and 140 mg/dl all the time. Now, you want to maintain that weight. You want to eat about 1,800 kilocalories, up another 300 from the previous diet in this chapter. Compared to the 1,200-kilocalorie diet, this may seem like a lot of food.

This plan provides 180 grams of carbohydrate, 135 grams of protein, and 60 grams of fat, providing roughly a 40:30:30 division of calories. You can use the recipes to create this diet as well, as shown in Table 3-4.

Exercise for prevention

A study published in the June 2007 edition of *Applied Physiology, Nutrition, and Metabolism* looked at numerous studies of the effect of exercise on the occurrence of diabetes. The study concluded that 30 minutes per day of moderate- or high-level physical activity can effectively and safely prevent type 2 diabetes in all populations.

Table 3-4	An 1,800-Kilocalorie Diet			
Meal	*Recipe*	*Carbs (g)*	*Protein (g)*	*Fat (g)*
Breakfast	Greek Omelet (Chapter 6)	8	20	13
	Two slices wheat toast	30	6	0
Lunch	Cauliflower Parmesan Soup (Chapter 8)	28	14	7
	3 oz. chicken	0	21	9
Dinner	Spit-Roasted Pork Loin (Chapter 14)	48	55	18
	Crispy Oatmeal Cookies (Chapter 16)	38.5	6	10.5
Total		**152.5**	**122**	**57.5**

This time, the plan is short 27.5 grams of carbohydrates, 13 grams of protein, and 2.5 grams of fat. You can make up the difference with snacks.

If you have type 2 diabetes, this plan is an excellent way for you to eat the right amount of calories. If you have type 1 diabetes, or you have type 2 and take insulin, you need to know the grams of carbohydrate in each meal in order to determine your insulin needs for that meal.

Checking Out Other Diets

If you go to the diet section of any large bookstore, you'll be overwhelmed by the choices. You'll find diets that recommend protein and no carbohydrate, carbohydrate and no protein, one type of carbohydrate and not another, all rice, all grapefruit, and on and on. How is it possible for all these diets, many of which are exactly the opposite of others on the same shelf, to actually work for you? The answer is they do and they don't. If you follow any diet closely, you'll lose weight. But will the weight stay off? That is the most difficult part (as we're sure you know).

In this section, we tell you about the most popular diets presently recommended by this or that brilliant "scientist." Which one do we recommend? None of them and all of them. If you find that you can get started losing weight successfully with one of these programs, go ahead and do it, but remember that in the end you want to eat a balanced diet that is low in fat and protein and uses carbohydrates that emphasize whole grains and fiber. And remember that you won't be successful without exercise.

Reduction of any source of calories — by reduction of carbohydrates, protein, or fat — has been shown to be equally effective.

The low carbohydrate group

These diets are based on the claim that carbohydrates promote hunger. By reducing or eliminating them, you lose your hunger as you lose your weight. The first of them, the Atkins Diet, promotes any kind of protein, including protein high in fat. Naturally, other diets were developed promoting very little carbohydrate but less fatty protein. Here are your choices:

- ✔ **Atkins Diet:** This plan allows any quantity of meats, shellfish, eggs, and cheese but doesn't permit high-carbohydrate foods like fruits, starchy vegetables, and pasta. Small quantities of the forbidden foods are added in later. The program does recommend exercise but doesn't suggest changes in your eating behavior.

- ✔ **South Beach Diet:** This diet restricts carbohydrates while the recommended proteins are low in fat, unlike the Atkins Diet. Daily exercise is an important component, but the plan doesn't suggest any changes in eating behavior. Over time some carbohydrate is reintroduced into the diet.

- ✔ **Ultimate Weight Solution:** This plan recommends a lot of protein, which naturally results in a reduction in carbohydrate. This program also advises you not to eat foods that are high in fat. Support groups in which you learn how to modify your eating behaviors are very important, and you're supposed to stay in these groups throughout your life. The plan also emphasizes regular exercise, such as walking.

- ✔ **Zone Diet:** In this diet, you have to balance your food intake into exact amounts of carbohydrate, protein, and fat. You're not permitted to eat high-carbohydrate and high-fat food. Regular exercise is recommended, but the plan doesn't suggest changes in your eating behavior. You have to continue with this balance throughout life to maintain your weight loss.

The portion control group

These diets recognize that it's not what you eat but how much you eat that determines your weight. They generally follow the recommendations of the government food guidelines. Here are some examples of portion control diets:

✔ **DASH Diet:** Here, the emphasis is on grains, fruits, and vegetables and restricting the amounts of fat. A further modification for those with high blood pressure recommends very little salt. Animal protein, such as meat, fish, and poultry, is limited. An exercise program is suggested but not defined. This diet suggests changes in eating behavior. It is a diet for life (and a very good one).

✔ **Jenny Craig:** This diet is balanced in terms of carbohydrates, protein, and fat but pushes its own food products, which can get expensive. You are directed to exercise by the counselor, who is an important (and costly) part of the program as well. To stay on this diet, you need its products lifelong.

✔ **Weight Watchers:** This plan uses a point system in which foods are given points according to the amount of fat, fiber, and calories in them. To get to and maintain a certain weight, you're given a daily number of points. As long as you stay within these points, you'll be successful. Therefore, foods that have large amounts of calories will use up your daily points quickly. The program suggests exercise and changes in your lifestyle.

A diet that emphasizes weight training

The Abs Diet is similar to the diets that recommend a balanced approach to eating, with carbohydrates that aren't refined and dairy and meat that are low in fat as the most suggested foods. However, the major emphasis in this diet is on a program called "Total Body Strength Training Workout" to build up the muscles. Changes in eating behavior aren't a large part of the program. To maintain weight loss, you must eat and exercise as the diet prescribes for your entire life.

More extreme diets

These diets require a level of participation that may be difficult for people who have a life. You really need to give your time and energy to staying on the diet. If you go away for a few weeks and stay within their program, you'll have some short-term success. But after you return home, sticking to the program gets difficult. Here are the two major programs currently available:

✔ **Dean Ornish Program:** This plan allows fruits, vegetables, and whole grains along with the leanest of meats and poultry. You can't eat processed foods or drink caffeine or alcohol, and you must avoid sugar, salt, and oil. Exercise is recommended as is help with eating behaviors. Meetings are an important part of this program, which you're supposed to follow for life.

✔ **Pritikin Eating Plan:** Whole grains, vegetables, and fruits are essential foods, and the diet allows almost no protein or fat. Exercise is a part of the program as is changing your lifestyle to promote better eating behaviors. You're expected to follow this program for life. Only Pritikin and a few others have been able to do this.

✔ **Paleo Diet:** This diet is supposedly based on the diet that our ancient ancestors ate — plenty of meat, nuts and vegetables but little of our modern agricultural foods like dairy, wheat, and legumes. But anyone who thinks that modern meat is anything like the meat that hunter-gatherers ate is sadly mistaken. Ancient people didn't suffer from our modern diseases of old age because they died young. This diet placed last among experts for *U.S. News & World Report* in both 2011 and 2012 with respect to health, weight loss, and ease of following.

✔ **Biggest Loser:** Based on a television show by the same name, this diet features small frequent meals consisting of lean protein, lowfat dairy, fruits, vegetables, whole grains, beans, and nuts. There is a huge amount of exercise associated with the diet. This program is very hard to sustain in real life.

With the exception of the DASH Diet, which is recommended by the U.S. government, none of the diets described in the preceding sections have long-term studies that show, convincingly, that they're better than any other. Each one of them has anecdotal evidence, meaning that one or two or ten people tell you how great they did on this or that diet. But you never hear from those who didn't do so great.

Chapter 4

Eating What You Like

. . . .

In This Chapter

▶ Having a plan for eating

▶ Enjoying your favorite ethnic foods

▶ Keeping the right ingredients at hand

▶ Choosing the best tools

▶ Making modifications for better diabetic control

▶ Getting through the holidays

. . . .

*H*aving diabetes doesn't mean you have to give up the foods that you grew up with and the foods you love the most. Some parts of every ethnic diet fit well in a diabetic regimen. You can find recipes to prove this premise in Part II of this book. You can also use all kinds of tricks to substitute good-for-you ingredients for those that won't help your diabetes. That's what this chapter is all about. Even foods that seemingly have no business on the plate of a diabetic can be enjoyed if eaten in small portions.

We wish we could eliminate the word "diet" from the diabetic vocabulary. The word implies taking something away or having to suffer somehow in order to follow it. This is not the case at all. You can eat great food and enjoy the taste of every ethnic variety, provided you concentrate on the amount of food and its breakdown into the sources of energy, keeping fats and carbohydrates in control. Perhaps the phrase "nutritional plan" would be better than "diet."

Stop dieting and start eating delicious foods. It may take a lot of willpower, but you can give up dieting if you try hard enough.

Staying True to Your Eating Plan

Creating an eating plan that provides the proper number of kilocalories from carbohydrate, protein, and fat (see Chapter 3) is particularly important when you have diabetes. After you know how much of each you need, you can translate those numbers into recipes and pick out the food that is the delicious end point of all the calculating. Make sure that your choices come from a variety of foods rather than eating the same thing over and over. You will be much more likely to stay on your program if you aren't bored with what you eat.

Before you cook, make sure that the recipes fit into your eating plan. If you have already eaten your carbohydrate portions for the day, make sure that the food you're about to eat has little carbohydrate in it. The same is true for protein and, of course, fat. If you think "moderation" as you make your meal plan, you'll keep to the portions you need to eat and no more.

Seasonal foods should play a primary role in your eating plan for several reasons:

✔ Seasonal foods are the freshest foods in the market.

✔ They are the least expensive foods.

✔ The recipes you can prepare with these fresh foods are some of the most delicious. The recipes in this book show the tremendous influence that fresh ingredients have had on the imaginations of the best chefs in the United States and Canada.

In addition, time is an important factor in your eating plan. You may not have a great deal of time to prepare your food, and some of the recipes in this book may take more time than you can spare. Choose the meals that fit into your schedule. But remember that after you've prepared a recipe a few times, preparation is much faster and easier. Consider the time you spend preparing delicious, healthy food as an investment in your well-being. Take the time to eat properly now so that later you won't have to spend your time being sick.

As a person with diabetes, especially if you have type 1 diabetes, you must figure the timing of your food in your eating plan. You need to eat when your medications will balance your carbohydrates. This process is much easier with the rapid-acting insulins, lispro and glulisine, but if you're still using regular insulin, you'll have to eat about 30 minutes after you take your shot.

Another essential part of your planning is what to do when you feel hungry but shouldn't eat. You can prepare a low-calorie snack for such occasions, or you can provide yourself with some diversion, such as a hobby, a movie, or, best of all, some exercise. Examples of low-calorie snacks are baby carrots, cherry tomatoes, a piece of fruit, and lowfat pudding.

Your diabetes medication may require you to have three meals a day, but if not, having three meals is still important. This approach spreads calories over the day and helps you avoid coming to a meal extremely hungry. Try not to skip breakfast, even though society doesn't encourage taking the time for this meal. Making your own lunch as often as possible gives you control over what you eat. The fast lunches served in restaurants may not provide the lowfat nutrition that you think you're getting. For example, salads are often covered with a lot of oil. It may be the right type of oil, but it still provides a lot of fat calories. And the portions may be greater than you think.

Enjoying the Best of Ethnic Cuisines

If you become diabetic, you don't have to give up the kinds of food you've always eaten. You can eat the same foods but decrease the portions, particularly if you're obese. People in ethnic groups who are normal in weight are doing two things that you need to do as well: eating smaller portions and keeping physically fit with exercise. Although many of these ethnic choices don't follow the Mediterranean pattern of eating, each has many healthful qualities. You don't have to adhere strictly to a Mediterranean diet — you can get some variety and still be healthy.

After you receive a diagnosis of diabetes, try to find a dietitian who treats many members of your ethnic group. This person will be best trained to show you how to keep eating what you love, while altering it slightly to fit your needs. The alteration may be no greater than simply reducing the amount of food that you eat each day. Or it may involve changing ingredients so that a high-fat source of energy is replaced by a lowfat energy source with no loss in taste.

Valuing African-American food

African-American food, sometimes called soul food, combines the food preferences and cooking methods of the African slaves with the available ingredients and available fuel found in the United States. Slow cooking with lots of vegetables and meats, eating lots of greens, combining fruits and meats in main dishes, and deep-frying meats and vegetables were cooking traditions brought to the United States. At the time, their foods, which contained too much fat, cholesterol, sugar, and salt, did not hurt the overworked and abused slaves because their daily energy needs were so great. Today, the more sedentary African-American population suffers from one of the highest incidences of obesity and diabetes, not to mention high blood pressure and the consequences of those diseases. As their energy needs fell, African Americans didn't reduce their calorie intake.

The term *soul food* also points to the central place of eating in the African-American population. In the slave quarters, the preparation and sharing of good food helped the slaves to maintain their humanity, helping those even less fortunate than themselves, who might have had no food at all. Because they had no other material possessions, food became the one symbol of wealth that wasn't taken from them. It also served as the focus of the creativity and artistic expression of the female slave.

But people don't have to abandon soul food. African-American cooks at home and chefs in restaurants have learned to use all the healthful ingredients, such as fruits, vegetables, and grains, with much smaller amounts of fat, sugar, and salt. They use spices in place of salt in very creative ways to bring out the taste of their fresh ingredients. The meats are leaner, and they use egg whites instead of the whole egg. They also avoid deep-frying as much as possible.

A new book published in March 2009 called *Vegan Soul Kitchen* by Bryant Terry (Da Capo Press) shows that you can make great soul food without animal protein or dairy.

The psychological implications of food in the African-American population means that changing from less healthy to more healthy food requires a change in mindset. African-American cooks can be just as creative or even more so with healthful ingredients. The use of less fat, less salt, and less sugar is essential, but other ingredients have to take their place. Quantities of food must be modified, and this may be the most difficult change, given the importance of food both as a symbol of wealth and for sharing. People must eat fewer cakes, pies, and cookies and find ways to creatively prepare fruit to take the place of sweet baked goods.

Appreciating Chinese food

When you think of Chinese food, you think rice. But China is such a huge place, and rice can't be grown everywhere. In the north, millet is used to make cereal. About 1500 B.C., wheat was introduced from West Asia. Vegetables such as soybeans and cucumbers were added to the rice, and occasionally a little bit of chicken or beef was added. Ginger became a favorite flavoring because it was so readily available.

The Thais gave chicken to China, and pork was already there, while Westerners brought sheep and cattle. The Chinese, mostly peasants, had little fuel and little cooking oil. Consequently, they learned to cut their food into very small pieces so it would cook rapidly, using little oil for their stir-frying.

Around 1000 A.D., because Buddhists, who made up a large part of the population, wouldn't eat meat, tofu or bean curd was introduced. The Chinese also learned to make long noodles from wheat and rice.

Chinese cuisine is generally healthful. It includes lots of vegetables, fruits, and seafood, while keeping sugar and desserts to a minimum. People with diabetes need to avoid eating too much rice. Chinese restaurants offer wonderful vegetable dishes, many with tofu as a protein source. You can go into any Chinese restaurant and find numerous dishes that have only vegetables with tofu.

When you cook Chinese food, use as little sugar and fat as possible, and steer clear of making deep-fried dishes.

Welcoming French food

French food is always associated with the term "haute cuisine," which means fine food prepared by highly skilled chefs. This kind of cooking derives from Italy and was introduced to France by Catherine de Medici. The French added their own subtle techniques to the methods of the Italians from Florence, adopting their use of truffles and mushrooms and preparing lighter sauces.

The French gave the world the technique of serving a series of dishes, one after the other, instead of a large buffet where people helped themselves to everything at once.

France has several distinct culinary regions:

- ✔ **The north:** Abundant forests provide game, and streams provide fish.
- ✔ **The central area:** The red wines provide the basis for much of the cooking.
- ✔ **The south:** Goose liver, truffles, and Roquefort cheese combine with Mediterranean olive oil, garlic, and tomatoes to produce the distinctive cuisine that is loved throughout the Western world, especially in its new lighter form. French food fits beautifully into the Mediterranean tradition of cooking.

You can go to Paris and find plenty of Mediterranean restaurants. French chefs — some of the best in the world — are geniuses at using whatever ingredients are at hand to make delicious meals.

Enjoying Italian food

Italian food reflects the history of Italy. Until 1870, Italy was divided into many different regions, with each one developing its own cuisine. Therefore, there is no one Italian food, but there are some common trends:

- ✔ The food of northern Italy features more wild game, such as deer and rabbits, along with some farm animals, such as beef, chickens, and goats. Seasonings include garlic, onions, rosemary, and bay leaf.

- ✔ In the south, much closer to the sea, seafood received much more emphasis. Southerners also developed some of the famous cheeses like ricotta and pecorino. It was here where the Italian staple, the artichoke, was first discovered and cultivated.

The invasions of Arabs from North Africa in southern Italy around 800 A.D. brought some of the foods that are now most typically thought of as Italian, things like melons, dates, rice, and lemons, but their major contribution was pasta. The Spanish gave the tomato to Italy, but the Italians took it over and made it their own.

Today, northern Italian cooking emphasizes cream and meat sauces. Rice dishes like risotto and polenta made from yellow corn are enjoyed along with gnocchi, a dumpling contributed by Germany.

As you move south, the olive becomes part of many dishes, along with wine for cooking. In southern Italy, the tomato is the basis of most cooking, particularly its use in pasta dishes. The cheeses mentioned earlier also are featured. The closeness of all parts of this region to the sea, as well as to the islands off the western coast, means that fish will be found in many meals.

These mouthwatering dishes aren't denied to the person with diabetes. The Mediterranean diet, with its emphasis on olive oil, has been shown to be healthy for your heart. One of the key changes you may need to make, however, is to reduce the amount of fat in your ingredients. Olive oil is a fat, and as you add more of it to your dishes, the calories climb rapidly. When Italians worked hard in the fields all day or traveled long distances to hunt or fish, they needed those extra calories to sustain them. But when was the last time you lifted a shovel or bagged a deer?

A second important step is reducing the size of your portion of pasta or risotto, whether you eat it at home or in the wonderful Italian restaurants (see Chapter 17 for more about eating healthy at restaurants). None of the recipes give you more than a cup of pasta or ⅔ cup of rice. Compare that with the usual 3 cups of pasta at a restaurant, and you quickly discover what changes you need to make.

On the other hand, the great fresh fruits and vegetables in Italian cooking are just what the doctor ordered, like the tomato, the artichoke, and the beans. These fit perfectly into the new emphasis of the federal food guidelines on fiber and reduction of fat. They also are the reason that Italian food is one of the easiest to convert to Mediterranean.

Top off your meal with a glass of Chianti from Tuscany. (Chapter 1 tells you about the benefits of alcohol.) But skip the rich Italian desserts or share a dessert with three other people. We don't think these changes will be a hardship. They take nothing away from the glory of Italian cooking.

Feasting on Mexican food

Mexican food comes from the Mayan Indians of the southeastern part of the country. They were hunters and fisherman, so their main sources of food were wild game, such as rabbit and turkey, and fish. Their diet also included beans and corn. The Aztecs later added chocolate, vanilla, honey, and chilies. After Spain conquered the country in 1521, the Spanish diet began to influence Mexican food. The Spanish brought livestock like cows and pigs and taught the Mexicans to make cheese and bread.

The type of Mexican food that has become so popular in the United States, the burrito, is a stuffed wheat tortilla. The Spanish brought in the wheat, so the burrito isn't exactly an indigenous food of Mexico. The Mexican tortilla is made of cornmeal, not wheat.

Mexico has been influenced by other colonial powers, including France, Portugal, all the surrounding islands in the Caribbean, West Africa, and South America.

As a result of the influences of other countries, Mexican food can be much more complex than the burrito. If you buy a small burrito, you get a fairly good combination of beans, chicken or beef, rice, and salsa, but you may also get your daily dose of salt in this single food. When you make your own, however, you can control the amount of salt.

The ingredients in a burrito, minus the high salt content, can make a nice meal in a hurry. When you make burritos, be sure to avoid cheese and excessive rice and watch out, especially, for the hot pepper.

Savoring Thai food

Thai food is a good choice for people with diabetes. It is cooked with little fat because stir-frying is the method of choice. Thai cooking keeps the meat, fish, and poultry to small quantities, thus providing taste rather than bulk, as in a Western diet. The dipping sauces have strong tastes, so they're used in very small quantities, minimizing the salt and sugar in the diet. Vegetables are eaten in larger quantities. At the end of the meal, Thais enjoy fruits like mango, pineapple, guava, and papaya, which provide fiber, vitamins, and minerals.

Thai food, like Italian food, is also the product of many influences. Westerners introduced milk into Thai cooking, and because coconut milk is so readily available, this became a staple of Thai dishes. The Chinese coming down from the north brought stir-frying with them, as well as noodles. Thanks to the Chinese, the five basic flavors of Asian cuisine — bitter, salt, sour, hot, and sweet — were established, and Thai meals use them as their basis for a balance of flavors. Dishes made with soy and ginger are a good example.

India brought curry dishes to Thailand, with coconut milk serving as an antidote to the hot spices in some of those curry dishes. The Thais have put their own delicious stamp on these curries, using a lot of green chile pepper, also given to them originally by Westerners.

Southern Thai food is usually hot and spicy, and fish is a major ingredient because the area is so close to the sea. However, you can always get dishes that aren't so spicy, and the subtle tastes of good Thai cooking have made it tremendously popular in the United States and throughout the world wherever Thais are found. Rice generally is part of the meal.

Most Thai dishes have garlic, a condiment that grows all over Thailand. Coconut milk, actually a combination of the coconut flesh and the liquid inside the coconut, is added to Thai curries and soups. Use the lowfat coconut milk if possible. Fish sauce, made by fermenting shrimp, salt, and water together, takes the place of soy sauce in Thai cooking.

In American Thai restaurants, a dish called pad thai has become a favorite entree. It means "Thai-style stir-fried noodles" and was brought to Thailand by the Chinese. When employment was low in Thailand after World War II, the government promoted noodle shops and stalls as a way of getting people back to work, and pad thai noodles became popular throughout the country. Thai immigrants brought the dish to the United States. It's not exactly representative of the finest Thai cuisine, but it's eaten so frequently in the United States that it must be considered when the diabetic has Thai food, particularly because the sauce often contains a lot of sugar and salt. A small portion of pad thai is fine for the person with diabetes, but leave at least half the serving for another day.

Thai food is so nutritious that there is little about it to warn the person with diabetes. As always, avoid large portions and too much rice. And be careful of the hot spices.

Relishing Latin American food

Although many countries make up Latin America, they have a number of similarities in the way they prepare food. Corn-based tortillas, tamales, tacos, pupusas, and arepas are found throughout Latin America. Salsas, guacamole, *chimichurri* (a mixture of parsley, olive oil, vinegar, cilantro, garlic, red pepper and cumin), *pico de gallo* (tomato, onion, jalapeño pepper, cilantro, green onion, and garlic), and other condiments make Latin American cuisine extremely flavorful but low in salt. Because all Latin American countries are on the water, seafood is a healthy staple. Rice and beans are eaten at most meals.

Although the prevalence of diabetes in Latin America has been low in the past, the increasing urbanization and decreasing physical activity is leading to many more people with the disease.

Eating the rest of the world's cuisine

Covering all the world's wonderful cuisines in detail isn't possible in this book. We tried to cover the most popular foods in the English-speaking world, but we could devote an entire book to every type of cuisine. We know that we left out delicious cuisines that many of you love from other countries, such as Greece, India, Guatemala, Costa Rica, Argentina, and Brazil. But we hope that you will still come away with a few general tips about these foods from around the world:

- ✔ You don't have to give up the foods you love because you have diabetes.
- ✔ Food is also love, sharing, social status, wealth (which it represented for slaves), and a lot more.
- ✔ You can avoid the empty calories in fatty, sugary desserts.
- ✔ The biggest problem is the large size of the portions. Try sharing or saving the food for another meal instead.
- ✔ A lot of exercise will reverse the damage of just about any dietary indiscretion.
- ✔ You can reduce the fat in your food, and it will still be delicious.
- ✔ You can reduce the salt and lower your blood pressure.

We want you to learn to eat to live — not live to eat. What you put in your mouth has a lot to do with your state of health, no matter where the food comes from.

Choosing from familiar foods

Esmeralda Cruz, a patient from a region of the Philippines called Pampanga, figured out how to successfully manage her diabetes without giving up the staples of her native cuisine. And good thing — her home is considered by many to be the culinary capital of the country. Esmeralda is a 46-year-old woman with type 2 diabetes, which has been diagnosed for five years. She is 5 feet, 2 inches tall and weighs 156 pounds. Her blood glucose averages 176 mg/dl, and she has a hemoglobin A1c of 8.6 percent.

Esmeralda followed a typical Filipino diet and gained at least 3 to 6 pounds each year for the last four years. She ate a lot of food fried in lard and too much rice for the calories and carbohydrate that are planned for her diet. She also tended not to trim the fat from the meat that she ate.

Her dietitian advised her to make modifications that would help her keep her diabetes in line without sacrificing the foods she loved. The dietitian recommended that Esmeralda do the following:

✔ Cut off visible fat from her meats

✔ Reduce the amount of frying and begin broiling and roasting instead

✔ Switch to canola oil in place of lard

✔ Reduce the amount of fat she used

✔ Eat less rice and choose low-glycemic types, like basmati

✔ Add more fish and poultry to her diet in place of meat

Esmeralda found that the alterations usually didn't affect the food's appeal. For example, one of her dishes, a pork dish called Tortung Babi, was made with three eggs, but reducing the number to two didn't diminish the taste.

After discovering how to modify her diet rather than giving up her native food, Esmeralda began to lose weight. She gradually lost 12 pounds over the next six months, and her blood glucose began to fall to the point that it averaged 132 mg/dl with a hemoglobin A1c of 6.9 percent. Because she made these changes for all members of her family, everyone has benefited.

Stocking Up with the Right Ingredients

Some common ingredients are used in many different recipes. Having them at hand is convenient, saving you needless trips to the market and more exposure to foods you don't need.

Some of the foods that belong in every kitchen or pantry (if you're a vegetarian, make the appropriate substitutions) include the following:

For the freezer:

Chicken breasts

Egg substitute

Frozen fruit

Fruit juice concentrate

Loaf of whole-wheat bread

For the pantry:

Canned fruit in fruit juice

Canned tomatoes

Canned tuna, salmon in water

Dried fruit, unsugared

Evaporated skim milk

Fat-free or reduced-fat salad dressing

Fresh garlic

Fruit spreads

Grains (rice, couscous)

Ketchup

Legumes (peas, beans, lentils)

Mustard

Nonfat dry milk

Nonstick cooking sprays

Oils (olive, canola, peanut)

Onions

Pasta (whole grain)

Pasta sauce

Peanut butter

Potatoes

Red and white cooking wines

Reduced-calorie mayonnaise

Reduced-sodium broths

Reduced-sodium soy sauce

Sugar-free cocoa mix

Tomato paste

Vinegars

Worcestershire sauce

For baking:

Baking powder

Baking soda

Cocoa powder

Cornstarch

Cream of tartar

Dry bread crumbs

Extracts (vanilla, lemon, almond)

Flour (all-purpose, whole-wheat)

Rolled oats

Semisweet chocolate

Sugar-free gelatin

Unflavored gelatin

Sweeteners:

Artificial sweeteners

Honey

Light maple syrup

Molasses

Sugar

Seasonings:

Dried herbs

Fresh herbs and spices

Pepper

Salt

With these ingredients, you're ready for just about any of the recipes in the book. The exceptions are exotic ingredients, such as in ethnic foods, that you can buy in specialty stores as you need them.

Prepare a list of these ingredients and make multiple copies so that you can check off what you need before you go to the market. Leave a little space for the perishables such as fresh fruits, vegetables, milk, meat, fish, and poultry. In the next chapter, we tell you more about the process of shopping for these ingredients.

Using the Right Tools

Just as you wouldn't try to bang in a nail with a shoe (especially with your foot inside), don't try to cook without the right tools. Spending a little more at the beginning pays huge dividends later on. For example, get the best set of knives you can afford. They make all cutting jobs much easier, and they last a long time. Buy good nonstick pans; they make cooking without oils much easier.

Here's the basic equipment that all kitchens should have in order to turn out delicious meals:

Chopping boards	Pots and pans
Food processor	Salad spinner
Knives	Scales
Measuring cups and spoons	Steamer with double boiler
Microwave	Thermometers (for roasts and turkey)
Mixer with dough hook	

Making Simple Modifications

You can make all kinds of simple modifications that will reduce calories and reduce the amounts of foods (such as those containing cholesterol) that you are trying to keep in check:

✔ Use skim milk instead of whole milk.

✔ Use fish or poultry and little red meat. If you eat occasional red meat, choose lower fat. Lower fat meats include lean beef, lean pork, and skinless white-meat poultry.

✔ Trim all visible fat off meats and poultry.

✔ Stay away from packaged luncheon meats, which tend to be high in fat and sodium.

✔ Select foods that are low in sodium and saturated fats (check the label on the food).

✔ Choose high-fiber foods like whole fruits, vegetables, and grains.

✔ Enjoy nonfat or reduced-fat yogurt instead of sour cream.

✔ Have dressings, sauces, and gravies served on the side.

✔ Substitute lentils and beans for meat, fish, and poultry.

✔ Replace butter with olive oil, herbs, spices, or lemon juice.

✔ Prepare foods by baking, broiling, and so on — any method other than frying.

Use your imagination to come up with your own unique ways to cut calories and fat.

Taking Holiday Measures

This is a particularly good heading for this section, because the key to getting through a holiday in good diabetic control is to control the portions of everything you eat during the holidays. Eating too much is easy.

If you encounter the "killer B," a buffet table, vow to make only one trip. You'll probably fill your plate with more food than you need, so plan to leave a large portion on the plate. Focus on the foods that you should eat and avoid high-fat and high-sugar foods, particularly desserts. Stick to fruits for high-fiber, low-calorie desserts.

If you're invited to a potluck dinner, make something that you know will work for your nutritional plan. You can certainly find something in this book that fits for you. These recipes have all been taste-tested and are delicious, so you don't have to think that you're bringing something inferior. We suggest that you have a snack before you go to a party so that you don't arrive feeling hungry.

Most important of all, try to forget the all-or-nothing mind-set. If you go off your nutritional plan once or twice, put the lapse behind you and get back to doing the things you know are right for you. The benefits will be immediate in the form of a general feeling of well-being and, of course, long-term in the fact that you won't develop the long-term complications of diabetes.

Chapter 5

How the Supermarket Can Help

In This Chapter

▶ Having a grocery shopping plan

▶ Reading the Nutrition Facts label

▶ Arming yourself to make good choices

*E*very trip to the market is an adventure. This chapter is about coping with the challenge of going grocery shopping without being lured into buying items that aren't good for your diabetes nutritional plan. But it's also about overcoming your natural desire to take home what you know isn't good for you.

You deserve the best, and that holds true for the food you eat as much as anything else. Of course, you could be like the man whose doctor told him that the best thing he could do for himself would be to get on a really good diet, stop chasing women, and stop drinking so much alcohol. The patient replied: "I don't deserve the best. What about second best?" We hope you won't settle for second best.

Going to the Market with a Plan

If you have a hobby, you've probably developed a series of steps by which you can accomplish your hobby in the most efficient manner, whether it's painting pictures or raising tomatoes. If you paint pictures, you certainly wouldn't start painting without deciding on a subject and buying the right paints, brushes, and canvas. If you raise tomatoes, you prepare the soil, add amendments such as manure, and buy the seeds or, more likely, the plants. You use a watering system as well as tomato cages to hold up your crop.

You should plan your excursion to the market in the same careful manner. Decide in advance what you need that complies with your nutritional plan. In Chapter 4, we give you a list of recommendations for the staples you should have at home. You can use those suggestions to make a shopping list to make sure that you purchase what you need. To that list, add the perishables that you'll use immediately, such as meat and poultry or fish, milk and other dairy products, and, of course, fruits and vegetables.

Eat something before you go to the market so that you aren't hungry as you walk down the aisles.

A market is like a huge menu set up to entice you. Most markets are set up in the same way. This setup is not by accident. It's arranged to encourage you to buy. What people buy on the impulse of the moment is often the most calorie-concentrated and expensive food that is least appropriate for them. You'll find that all the perishable food is arranged around the perimeter of the market. The high-calorie foods are in the aisles in the middle of the store. Unless you want to take the long way around, you must go through those aisles to get to the meat, milk, fruit, and vegetables. You pass the loose candies, the cookies, the high-sugar cereals, and all the other no-nos. If you prepare a list and buy only from the list, you won't purchase any of those foods. Walking into the market hungry and without a list is dangerous for your health.

Sometimes the market employs a person who is trained to help people with medical conditions make the best selections. Check with your market to find out whether such a person is on staff, and spend some time touring the aisles with him or her. You'll get some valuable insights that will make handling a shopping trip easier.

Some keys to shopping the market most effectively include the following:

- ✔ Shop at the same market each time.
- ✔ Shop as seldom as you can.
- ✔ Go to the market when it is not crowded.
- ✔ Don't walk every aisle.
- ✔ Don't be tempted by free samples. They're usually high in calories to appeal to your taste buds.
- ✔ If you bring your kids (not advisable) to the store, make sure that they aren't hungry.
- ✔ Be especially careful in the checkout lane, where stores force you to run through a gauntlet of goodies — none of which are good for you.

The bakery

You can really make a dent in your diet in the bakery section, where all the desserts are on display. These foods usually contain too much fat and carbohydrate; however, you don't have to give up all your "treats." The key is to figure a rich dessert into your meal plan, but only on an occasional basis. Remember to keep the portion small, in any case.

Muffins and pastries are usually high in fat, but in deference to the popular belief that fat makes us fat, stores now sell lowfat muffins and pastries. The problem is that these still contain many calories, so don't overdo it. Try a smaller portion or share your muffin with a friend. A popular choice is angel food cake, but watch out because, even though it's totally fat-free, it's filled with kilocalories. You can enjoy a small portion.

Select breads that have at least 2 grams of fiber per slice and whole-grain breads. Bagels and English muffins should be whole-grain as well. Don't forget that they're usually too large, so plan on eating a serving of half or less. (That goes for any bread.) If you eat too much, you'll consume too many calories.

Produce

Fruits and vegetables are in the produce section. These make up half of your plate (see Chapter 2 for more on MyPlate). Stores continue to offer the usual apples, pears, and bananas, but today they stock more fruits and vegetables that you may never have seen before. Here is where you can add some real variety to your diet. Try some of these new items, and you may discover that you can substitute them for the cakes, pies, and other concentrated calorie foods that you now eat. For example, you may find that you like some of the new varieties of melons, which are sweet and have a great texture.

The other benefit to trying new fruits and vegetables is that you get a variety of vitamins and minerals from the different sources. Each differently colored vegetable provides different vitamins, so pick out a variety of colors.

To prolong their season, you can freeze some of the fruits, especially the berries, and use them as you need them.

Remember that dried fruits have very concentrated carbohydrate and should be used sparingly.

Root vegetables need no refrigeration but must be kept in a cool, dry place. Most of the other vegetables must go in the refrigerator.

The dairy case

At the dairy case, you can make some very positive diet modifications. Go for the lowest fat content you can eat, but don't neglect the dairy part of MyPlate. That's where you get calcium. Try to find lowfat cheeses, yogurt, and cottage cheese. Go for 1 percent or even skim milk if possible.

The deli counter

A deli counter offers luncheon meats and prepared foods. Recent studies show that these processed meats are dangerous to your health. These foods often contain a lot of salt and fat. You probably want to avoid most of the foods in this area (with the exception of prepared chicken, which is often spit-roasted and very tasty). Even the lowfat meats in this section are rich in salt. The pickled foods may also contain a great deal of salt, despite being low in calories and free of fat.

If you choose salads from this area, pick out those that contain oil instead of cream. Don't be afraid to ask a deli employee about the exact ingredients in these prepared foods. In some cases, lower-fat versions are available. People often prefer fatty foods — and the grocery obviously wants people to buy the food — so the market caters to those preferences.

The fresh meat and fish counter

The fresh meat and fish counter provides some good choices for your protein needs. At the meat counter, buy no more than a normal serving for each member of the family. Just because the meat attendant has cut a 12-ounce piece of swordfish doesn't mean that you have to buy the whole thing. You are entitled to get just the piece you want. For convenience, you can get two servings at one time if you know you have the willpower to save the second serving for another meal. Ask the attendant to cut the fish in half so you aren't tempted to eat the whole thing.

Don't forget that lentils and other legumes can provide protein as well.

Try to buy skinless poultry to eliminate a major source of the fat in chicken. You may have to cook it a shorter time, or you can barbecue the chicken using an indirect method (place the coals along the sides of the chicken rather than underneath). The chicken will be much juicier and not dried out.

Try to eat fish at least twice a week because of the positive effect it has on blood fats. Remember that a "fatty" fish such as salmon is good for you but adds extra fat calories.

The fresh meat and fish counter usually offers breaded or battered fish to make your life easier; you only have to put it in the oven. The problem is that the breading or batter often contains too much butter, fat, and salt. Ask the person serving you for a list of the ingredients in the breading or batter. Or better yet, skip the prepared fish and head for the fresh. If you notice a very fishy smell, then the fish is not very fresh.

Frozen foods and diet meals

When the season for your favorite fresh fruits and vegetables is over, the frozen food section may stock these items. However, because markets now often bring in more varieties of fresh food from all over the world year-round, you may not need to turn to frozen products as much.

Food manufacturers are producing a variety of frozen foods, which you can heat in the microwave oven. These meals are often high in fat and salt, however. Be sure to read the food label, which we explain later in this chapter. Avoid frozen foods mixed with cream or cheese sauces.

Diet meals can be a good choice if you want to save time in preparation. The frozen diet meals are low in calories and often low in salt and fat as well. Most diet meals have no more than 350 kilocalories and usually taste good. If you have type 1 diabetes and need to count carbohydrates, they're listed on the box.

Healthy Choice, Lean Cuisine, and Weight Watchers are the three main makers of diet meals, all of which can be counted on for low calories and good taste. Healthy Choice is the lowest in salt. Grocery stores usually have one brand or another on sale, so you can choose the least expensive brand when you shop.

Are frozen diet foods a good choice for you? Many of our patients complain that they lack time to prepare the "right" foods. For those people, prepared diet meals work very well. For the person who likes to involve him- or herself in food preparation — for example, people who bought this book for the wonderful recipes — this is not the way to go.

Low-carbohydrate foods are also being made by many of the food manufacturers. See our discussion of the various types of diets in Chapter 3 for ways that these foods can fit in your nutrition plan.

Canned and bottled foods

Canned and bottled foods can be healthful and can help you quickly make recipes calling for ingredients such as tomato sauce. Check the Nutrition Facts label (covered later in this chapter) to determine what kind of liquid a food is canned in. Oil adds a lot of fat calories, so look for the same food canned in water.

The case against sugar keeps getting stronger. Not only does it lead to weight gain, but it increases blood pressure, raises the risk of gout, causes liver damage, and accelerates the aging process. It's not the sugar in fruits and vegetables but the *added sugar* that the manufacturer adds during processing and that you add to your diet in the form of sugar, syrup, honey, high-fructose corn syrup, and molasses. Don't buy canned and bottled foods with added sugar, and keep your additions to a minimum.

Canned vegetables often contain too much salt, so look for low-salt varieties. Canned fruits often contain too much sweetener, so you're better off with fresh if possible.

Watch for this marketing trick: Stores often display higher-priced canned foods at eye level and lower priced products on lower shelves. Also, store brands are often less expensive and just as good as name brands.

Bottled foods include fruit juice drinks, which are high in sugar and low in nutrition. You're better off drinking pure fruit juice rather than a juice drink diluted with other ingredients.

The same principle is true for bottled and canned soda, which has no nutritional value and lots of calories. Substitute water for this expensive and basically worthless food that really doesn't quench your thirst (soft drinks often leave an aftertaste, especially the diet drinks). Try adding lemon or lime to your water or use the flavored calorie-free water drinks.

You can find lowfat or fat-free salad dressing and mayonnaise in this area. Better yet, try using mustard and some of the other condiments to spice up your salads without adding many calories.

The best choices for snacks

You probably frequently feel like eating a little something between meals. Your choice of foods may make the difference between weight gain and weight control, between high blood glucose levels and normal levels. Here are the best selections to choose as you make your way around the supermarket:

- ✔ **Baked chips:** Avoid fried chips, which add lots of fat calories. An ounce of baked chips amounts to 110 kilocalories.
- ✔ **Flavored rice cakes:** These items are filling without adding too many calories.
- ✔ **Fruit and fig bars:** These items can satisfy hunger without many kilocalories. A couple of Fig Newtons, for example, will set you back only 120 kilocalories.

- ✔ **Lowfat granola:** Watch out for regular granola, which is high in calories. Depending on the brand, ½ cup of lowfat granola contains 220 to 250 kilocalories.

- ✔ **Plain popcorn:** If you prepare it in an air-popping machine or a microwave oven, it contains only 30 kilocalories per cup and is free of salt and fat.

- ✔ **Raisins and other dried fruit:** Stick to small portions. A quarter of a cup of raisins is only 130 kilocalories.

- ✔ **Fresh fruit:** A typical serving is 60 to 80 kilocalories.

- ✔ **Fresh vegetables:** Carrots, celery, and so forth.

The preceding list should give you enough choices to satisfy your hunger without wrecking your diabetic control.

Taking advantage of farmer's markets

One of the best innovations of the last decade has been the proliferation of farmer's markets, which bring together produce from local farmers with extremely fresh fish and poultry. Take it from us: There is nothing tastier than an heirloom tomato just picked by the farmer and sold to you that day. Many of the farmers have made their farms organic, which means their produce is free from harmful pesticides. Although farmer's markets often include bakeries, you can easily walk past those stands. If you do stop there, opt for delicious, freshly baked whole-wheat breads — they're wonderful on your Mediterranean diet.

The vegetables at farmer's markets have just been picked and are at the peak of their taste — unlike those in the supermarkets, which are grown more for their lasting qualities than their taste. The same is true of the fruits. Compare farmer's market strawberries with supermarket strawberries, and you'll never buy supermarket strawberries again.

The produce you find there can cost a bit more than produce in the supermarkets (but often they cost less!). If the produce does cost more, the difference is worth every penny. Plus, you're supporting local growers and getting the best that money can buy. The produce may be very seasonal, but who says that melons should be enjoyed in January?

The other noteworthy thing about the farmer's markets is the general air of festivity to be found there. Everyone is smiling! Farmers are happy to explain how they grow the produce and which ones they most recommend. If by chance you buy something and it isn't up to your standard, the farmer will likely replace it the next week or give you your money back. And you can taste everything! It's okay to go to the farmer's market hungry — the fruits and vegetables you taste won't hurt you!

Deciphering the Mysterious Food Label

Most packaged foods have a food label known as the Nutrition Facts label, which isn't really mysterious if you know how to interpret it. It was designed to be understood. Figure 5-1 shows a typical food label. The contents of the Nutrition Facts label are regulated by the Food and Drug Administration.

Figure 5-1:
A Nutrition
Facts food
label.

Nutrition Facts

Serving Size 1/2 cup (113g)
Servings Per Container 4

Amount Per Serving

Calories 120   Calories from Fat 15

	% Daily Value
Total Fat 1.5g	3%
Saturated Fat 1.0g	5%
Cholesterol 10mg	3%
Sodium 290mg	12%
Total Carbohydrate 15g	5%
Dietary Fiber 0g	
Sugars 14g	
Protein 10g	10%

© John Wiley & Sons, Inc.

The label in Figure 5-1 is from a 1-pound container of cottage cheese with fruit. You can find the following information on the label:

- **Serving Size:** The serving size is the portion of the total contents that makes up one serving. Most packaged foods serve more than one person so don't be fooled.

- **Servings Per Container:** At ½ cup, this container holds 4 servings.

- **Calories:** The number of kilocalories in a serving — in this case, 120 kilocalories.

- **Calories from Fat:** The number of fat kilocalories in each serving.

- **% Daily Value:** The nutrient amounts appear in grams or milligrams and also as % Daily Value. The % Daily Value refers to the percentage of the daily value for a person on a 2,000-kilocalorie-per-day diet. *Note:* If you're overweight, 2,000 kilocalories are more than you should eat, so reduce your serving portion appropriately.

- **Total Fat:** The total fat is 1.5 grams, of which 1.0 is saturated fat. The fact that there's less than 3 grams of fat allows the producer to refer to this product as *lowfat.*

✔ **Saturated Fat:** The amount of the fat in each serving that is saturated.

✔ **Cholesterol:** This food provides little cholesterol. Therefore, the producer could call it "low cholesterol" because that term applies if the product provides less than 20 milligrams of cholesterol and 2 grams or less of saturated fat per serving (see Chapter 2 for more information).

✔ **Sodium:** At 290 milligrams of sodium, this food provides 12% of the sodium allowed in a 2,000-kilocalorie-a-day diet.

✔ **Total Carbohydrate:** As a person with diabetes, you need to know the grams of carbohydrate in a serving, both to fit it into your nutritional plan and to determine insulin needs if that is what you take.

✔ **Dietary Fiber:** This food provides no fiber, so all the carbohydrate is digestible. If fiber were present, you could subtract the fiber grams from the total grams of carbohydrate to get the actual grams from carbohydrate absorbed.

✔ **Sugars:** The fact that 14 of the 15 grams of carbohydrate come from sugar means that the sugar will be absorbed rapidly.

✔ **Protein:** As a person with diabetes, you need to be aware of the grams of protein in a portion. The figure for % Daily Value doesn't help you in planning your diet.

✔ **Vitamins and Minerals:** Usually, the label provides the % Daily Value for vitamin A, vitamin C, calcium, and iron. Some food labels follow that information with a list of ingredients, but this information isn't required as part of the Nutrition Facts label.

The Food and Drug Administration wants to update the Nutrition Facts label in the following ways:

✔ Require information about "added sugars."

✔ Update daily values for sodium, fiber, and vitamin D.

✔ Add potassium levels to the label.

✔ Remove Calories from Fat from the label because the type of fat is more important.

✔ Change serving size to reflect how people eat and drink today.

✔ Require that packaged foods eaten in one sitting like large bottles of soda be labeled as one serving.

✔ Put per-serving and per-package labels on packages that may be consumed in one sitting.

✔ Make calories and serving sizes more prominent.

✔ Shift the % Daily Values to the left to give them more emphasis.

These changes will help consumers understand how much they're eating.

Making Good Choices

Thanks to the food labels, you can choose foods that are lower in calories, lower in fat, and have more nutritional value. You can compare foods next to one another and choose the healthier item. For example:

- ✔ Smart Balance has only 60 kcal per tablespoon while I Can't Believe It's Not Butter has 90 kcal per tablespoon.

- ✔ Uncle Ben's Fast and Natural Whole Grain Instant Brown Rice has 170 kcal per cup while Uncle Ben's Ready Rice Whole Grain Brown has 240 kcal per cup.

- ✔ Nature's Own Double Fiber Wheat Bread has 100 kcal per 2 slices while Arnold Double Fiber Whole Wheat Bread has 200 kcal per 2 slices.

- ✔ Annie's Naturals Buttermilk Dressing has 60 kcal in 2 tablespoons while Ken's Steak House Thousand Islands Dressing has 140 kcal per 2 tablespoons.

- ✔ Campbell's Healthy Request Condensed Chicken Noodle Soup has 60 kcal per cup while Campbell's Condensed Vegetable Soup has 100 kcal per cup.

We could go on and on like this, but you get the idea. There are tons of good choices that have fewer calories and often more fiber, vitamins, and minerals than the bad choices. You just need to spend a little time and look at the labels. The less the food is processed, the better it is for you.

Be sure you are comparing one serving to one serving. If you compare one serving to two servings, the larger item is bound to have many more calories.

Part II
Healthy Recipes That Taste Great

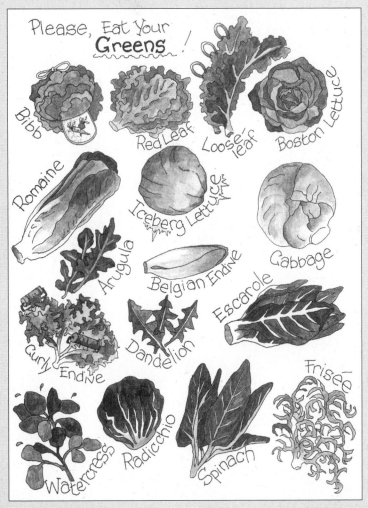

Illustration by Elizabeth Kurtzman

Find out how the Mediterranean lifestyle can help with diabetes in a free article at www.dummies.com/extras/diabetescookbook.

In this part . . .

- Get off to a good start with appetizers.
- Sip your nutrition with soup.
- Get enough protein from grains and legumes.
- Fill up with vegetables.
- Prepare fish for taste and health.
- Enjoy delicious fruit for dessert.

Chapter 6

The Benefits of Breakfast

In This Chapter

▶ Updating classic breakfast mainstays

▶ Baking muffins, biscuits, and quick breads

▶ Making the most of your egg choices

A big part of keeping your blood sugar steady is eating regularly. Typically, the longest break without food during a day comes at night. While your body rests and revitalizes itself, your blood glucose level takes a nosedive. Start your day the right way with a healthy balanced breakfast each and every day.

Choose a quick scrambled egg and whole-wheat toast if you're in a hurry. But brush up on the recipes in this chapter for a change of pace. By planning ahead, you can make a delicious breakfast that's anything but boring.

Understanding Diabetic Breakfasts

Breakfast is a critical meal for a diabetic. Getting your day off to a steady, balanced start sets you up for success the rest of the day. Check out Chapter 4 if you need help planning your meals for the day based on your individual needs. The following sections can help you make the right breakfast choices.

Figuring out which fruit is right for you

Fruit doesn't have to be a dirty word for a diabetic. While it's true that fruit is full of natural sugars and your body processes them quickly, you don't have to (and shouldn't) mark them off your list completely.

Whole fruit, rather than juice, is a better choice for diabetics. The fiber and skin in whole fruit slow down the digestion of the fruit, resulting in a more gradual rise in your blood sugar level.

Here's a list of fruits with a lower glycemic index (which we discuss in more detail in Chapter 2):

✔ Apples

✔ Apricots

✔ Blueberries

✔ Cherries

✔ Grapefruit

✔ Kiwis

✔ Strawberries

And just for balance, here are a few fruits with a higher glycemic index:

✔ Cantaloupe

✔ Dates

✔ Pineapple

✔ Raisins

✔ Watermelon

Just because a fruit has a higher glycemic index doesn't mean you can't eat it. Just take it into consideration when you plan when you eat it and what you eat with it. Plan to eat smaller amounts of high-GI foods.

Putting together protein-packed punches

Eggs aren't the only breakfast protein. In fact, many diabetics must limit their intake of cholesterol, and eggs are an easy target for removal. (Check out "Enjoying Egg-ceptional Dishes," later in this chapter, for smart ways to include eggs at breakfast.) Consider other nontraditional choices when you're making your breakfast changes. Here's a list of protein-rich foods that might make a good addition to your breakfast table:

- 1 turkey hot dog wrapped in a whole-wheat tortilla

- 1 ounce boiled shrimp with cocktail sauce

- 2 tablespoons of peanut butter on whole-wheat toast

- 1 slice turkey wrapped around lowfat string cheese

- 4-ounce grilled chicken breast

- ¼ cup cottage cheese with diced grape tomatoes

- Nonfat plain Green yogurt with milled flax, a few almonds, and berries

- Steel-cut oats with protein powder mixed in

- A smoothie with 8 ounces milk, 2 tablespoons nut butter, and frozen banana

Starting with Whole-Grain Goodness

When you received your diagnosis of diabetes, maybe you thought your days of eating waffles and pancakes were over. Although starting the morning off with pancakes dripping with butter and maple syrup is probably not in your current eating plan, you can still enjoy relatively sweet treats in the morning, especially if you use whole grains.

Refined grains are processed to remove the bran and the hull, and along with them, up to 90 percent of the nutrients, including vitamins E and B. Whole grains have a lower glycemic index than refined grains. So whole grains are less likely to send your blood glucose soaring and then dipping. The protein, fat, and fiber in whole grains slow their absorption into the bloodstream. In addition, whole grains make you feel fuller and stay fuller longer.

Read labels carefully to ensure that the food you're getting is made from whole grains. Don't just look for "wheat" bread; make sure it says "whole wheat." Some manufactures add caramel color or molasses to refined flour and sell the bread as "wheat bread," potentially confusing hopeful healthy eaters. Choose the food with more fiber.

Warm Blueberry Oats

Prep time: 5 min • **Cook time:** 3 min • **Yield:** 2 servings

Ingredients	Directions
1 cup rolled oats 2 cups water	*1* In a microwave-safe bowl, combine the oats and water. Microwave on high for 3 minutes.
2 teaspoons honey 1 cup fresh blueberries	*2* Remove the bowl from the microwave and stir in the honey and then the blueberries.

Per serving: Kcalories 218 (From Fat 25); Fat 3g (Saturated 0g); Cholesterol 0mg; Sodium 6mg; Carbohydrate 43g (Dietary Fiber 6g); Protein 7g.

Whole-Wheat Waffles

Prep time: 90 min • **Cook time:** 16 min • **Yield:** 4 servings

Ingredients	Directions
1 cup evaporated skim milk **1 teaspoon active dry yeast** **1 cup whole-wheat flour** **½ teaspoon orange zest** **⅛ teaspoon vanilla extract** **2 packets Splenda** **Nonstick cooking spray**	*1* Warm the milk and dissolve the yeast in it. In a bowl, mix the yeast mixture with the flour, orange zest, vanilla, and Splenda. Let sit, covered, at room temperature for 1½ hours. *2* Using a waffle maker coated with nonstick cooking spray, prepare the waffles, following the manufacturer's instructions.

Per serving: Kcalories 157 (From Fat 7); Fat 1g (Saturated 0g); Cholesterol 3mg; Sodium 76mg; Carbohydrate 30g (Dietary Fiber 4g); Protein 9g.

Tip: Instead of syrup, serve these beauties with Warm Pineapple Salsa. You can find the recipe in Chapter 7.

Tip: Skip the butter because these waffles are delicious without it. If you don't feel like you can go cold turkey, look for a spread, such as Brummel and Brown Yogurt Spread or Smart Balance Buttery Spread, that contains no trans fat.

Blueberry and Almond Pancakes

Prep time: 10 min • **Cook time:** 5–7 min • **Yield:** 4 servings (16 pancakes total)

Ingredients	*Directions*
½ cup all-purpose flour	**1** In a bowl, combine the all-purpose flour, whole-wheat flour, apple juice concentrate, baking powder, and salt; set aside.
¾ cup whole-wheat flour	
2 teaspoons apple juice concentrate	
2 teaspoons baking powder	**2** In another bowl, combine the applesauce, milk, almond extract, egg whites, blueberries, and almonds; stir well. Add the flour mixture. Stir until you achieve a fairly smooth batter consistency, approximately 2 minutes. Feel free to leave a few lumps, because overmixing can result in a tougher finished pancake.
¼ teaspoon salt	
1½ teaspoons unsweetened applesauce	
1¼ cups lowfat milk	
⅛ teaspoon almond extract	**3** Coat a large skillet with the cooking spray; place over medium heat until hot. Spoon ¼ cup batter for each pancake. When bubbles form on top of the pancakes, turn them over. Cook until the bottom of each pancake is golden brown.
3 egg whites, or 6 tablespoons egg substitute	
¾ cup fresh blueberries, or frozen berries, thawed	
1 tablespoon almond slivers, crushed	
Nonstick cooking spray	

Per serving: Kcalories 209 (From Fat 21); Fat 2g (Saturated 1g); Cholesterol 3mg; Sodium 419mg; Carbohydrate 38g (Dietary Fiber 4g); Protein 10g.

Stocking Up on Baked Goods

Having diabetes doesn't mean you have to deprive yourself of the ease (and deliciousness!) of grabbing a muffin, biscuit, or slice of quick bread. Plan ahead and keep some of these heart-healthy handfuls on hand for breakfast on the go.

We help you ease into using whole grains in this section by using a blend of all-purpose (white) flour and whole-wheat flour. You can find whole-wheat flour in the baking aisle in just about any grocery store.

Zucchini Bread

Prep time: 12 min • **Cook time:** 45–60 min • **Yield:** 18–20 servings

Ingredients	Directions
Nonstick cooking spray	*1* Preheat the oven to 350 degrees. Spray 2 loaf pans, 9 x 5 inches or 8 x 5 inches, with nonstick spray.
1½ cups whole-wheat flour	
1½ cups all-purpose flour	*2* In a large bowl, combine the whole-wheat flour, all-purpose flour, sugar, pecans, cinnamon, baking soda, and baking powder.
1 cup sugar	
½ cup chopped pecans	
1 teaspoon cinnamon	*3* In another bowl, combine the egg whites, applesauce, and buttermilk. Mix in the zucchini. Then combine with the flour mixture.
1 teaspoon baking soda	
¼ teaspoon baking powder	
6 egg whites	*4* Pour the mixture into the loaf pans. Bake 45 minutes to 1 hour. Insert a toothpick in the center of the loaf. When it comes out clean, the bread is done. Cool in the pan for 5 minutes and then cool completely on a wire rack.
1 cup applesauce	
½ cup buttermilk	
2½ cups grated zucchini	

Per serving: Kcalories 139 (From Fat 22); Fat 3g (Saturated 0g); Cholesterol 0mg; Sodium 92mg; Carbohydrate 26g (Dietary Fiber 2g); Protein 4g.

Tip: Don't bother peeling the zucchini before grating it. Just wash it and grate away. Double the recipe and freeze the second loaf. You'll definitely use it!

Sweet Potato Biscuits

Prep time: 25 min • **Cook time:** 12 min • **Yield:** 6 servings (12 biscuits total)

Ingredients	Directions
1 cup all-purpose flour	***1*** Preheat the oven to 425 degrees. In a bowl, combine the all-purpose flour, whole-wheat flour, baking powder, baking soda, and salt. With a pastry blender or fork, work in the butter until the mixture is coarse.
1 cup whole-wheat flour	
2½ teaspoons baking powder	
¼ teaspoon baking soda	***2*** In another bowl, combine the buttermilk and mashed sweet potatoes. Add to the flour mixture and mix until just moistened.
¼ teaspoon salt	
2 tablespoons butter	
½ cup buttermilk	***3*** Transfer the dough to a lightly floured surface. Knead 2 or 3 times, until smooth (see Figure 6-1). Roll out the dough ½-inch thick. Using a 2-inch biscuit cutter, dipped in flour, cut out 12 rounds.
⅔ cup mashed cooked sweet potatoes	
Nonstick cooking spray	***4*** Coat a baking sheet with the cooking spray. Arrange the rounds on the baking sheet. Bake for 12 minutes, until golden brown.

Tip: Use White Lily brand flour and whole-wheat pastry flour for more-tender biscuits.

Per serving: Kcalories 208 (From Fat 41); Fat 5g (Saturated 3g); Cholesterol 11mg; Sodium 333mg; Carbohydrate 37g (Dietary Fiber 4g); Protein 6g.

Figure 6-1: Knead dough by pressing, folding, and rotating it.

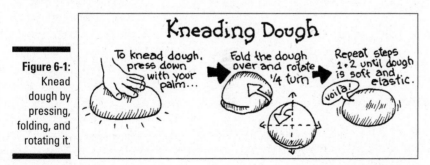

Kneading Dough

To knead dough, press down with your palm...

Fold the dough over and rotate ¼ turn

Repeat steps 1 + 2 until dough is soft and elastic.

voila!

Illustration by Elizabeth Kurtzman

Enjoying Egg-ceptional Dishes

Choosing eggs gives you a protein power punch to start your day. This simple food is an ideal source of protein, containing all essential amino acids. Eggs are also a source of B complex vitamins, vitamin A, vitamin D, vitamin E, selenium, and zinc. However, egg yolks also contain a significant amount of cholesterol. Consequently, low-cholesterol diets restrict the number of eggs allowed each week. People with diabetes should limit their eggs to a couple per week for the same reason.

One great way to enjoy eggs but limit your cholesterol is to enjoy egg whites or use a combination of whole eggs and egg whites. The egg yolk (the yellow center) contains the dreaded cholesterol, so limiting your intake of yolks may be enough to keep egg whites on your list.

Baking egg pies and quiches

These baked breakfast egg dishes are a great way to make delicious, healthy meals for a group. They're a great choice for elegant brunch entertaining or a weekday when you have a little extra time. Alternately, you can make a pie or quiche, cool it completely, and then cut it into individual servings and freeze them for later.

Broccoli and Cheese Pie

Prep time: 20 min • **Cook time:** 30 min • **Yield:** 4 servings

Ingredients	Directions
Nonstick cooking spray	*1* Preheat the oven to 350 degrees. Coat a 9-inch pie pan with the cooking spray.
1 cup fresh broccoli, small florets	
½ cup low-sodium chicken broth	*2* In a saucepan, cook the broccoli with the chicken broth, uncovered, over medium heat, stirring, until all liquid has evaporated, about 10 minutes. Transfer to a bowl and chill in the refrigerator for 5 minutes.
2 egg whites, lightly beaten	
1 whole egg, lightly beaten	*3* In another bowl, whisk together the egg whites and egg. Add the broccoli, milk, cheese, and pepper.
1 cup skim milk	
1 cup shredded cheddar cheese	*4* Pour the mixture into the pie pan and bake, uncovered, for 30 minutes, and check with a toothpick for doneness. (The pie may need to bake for up to 45 minutes.) Remove from the oven and cool.
¼ teaspoon pepper	

Per serving: Kcalories 171 (From Fat 99); Fat 11g (Saturated 7g); Cholesterol 85mg; Sodium 268mg; Carbohydrate 5g (Dietary Fiber 1g); Protein 13g.

Tuscan Quiche

Prep time: 30 min • **Cook time:** 40 min • **Yield:** 6 servings

Ingredients	Directions
24 ounces extra firm tofu 8 ounces vegan soy mozzarella	*1* Make the filling. Chop tofu and mozzarella into cubes, place in a food processor, and mix until smooth. Place the mixture in a bowl and chill.
1 tablespoon olive oil ½ cup chopped fine garlic ½ cup chopped fine shallots 1 16-ounce can quartered artichoke hearts (in water) 1 pound blanched chopped spinach Salt and pepper to taste 2 tablespoons nutritional yeast 1 tablespoon granulated onion 1 tablespoon granulated garlic	*2* Meanwhile, add the olive oil, garlic, and shallots in a sauté pan. Sauté until ingredients are translucent. Add the artichoke hearts and spinach to the pan and mix well. Season to taste with salt and pepper. Allow this mixture to cool and then add it to the tofu mixture. Add in the dry spices and stir well. Check for seasoning. Place the mixture in the fridge until ready to use.
	3 Meanwhile, preheat the oven to 350 degrees. On a cutting board, cut margarine into flour and salt. Quickly add in the water, one tablespoon at a time, until the mixture forms into a solid dough mass. Roll the dough out to a half-inch thick pancake, and then drape it over an oiled 9-inch pie pan, tucking in all the corners. Bake for 15 minutes or until golden brown. Remove from the oven, cool.
2 tablespoons soy margarine 1 cup whole-wheat pastry flour Kosher salt	*4* Place the tofu mixture into the cooked pie shell. Smooth out the mixture and return to the oven for 25 minutes. Remove from the oven.
4 tablespoons ice cold water	*5* Cool until the center is firm; slice and serve.

Per serving: Kcalories 380 (Calories from Fat 159); Fat 18g (Saturated 2g); Cholesterol 0mg; Sodium 606mg; Carbohydrate 32g (Dietary Fiber 7g); Protein 30g.

Tip: Look for nutritional yeast in the bulk section of your local natural food store. It's a complete protein and high in vitamin B-12. With its strong, nutty, cheesy flavor, it's used as a cheese substitute.

Trying your hand at omelets and frittatas

Omelets and *frittatas* (open-faced omelets) are among the best and easiest ways to get a burst of protein to start your day. In this section, we give you several flavorful recipes to keep your taste buds hopping.

Facing facts about feta cheese

If you haven't tried this terrific Greek cheese, here's your chance. It's a soft, salty cheese that has a tangy bite. It crumbles very easily, and is an easy addition to salads, eggs, or stuffed in olives. The commercially available variety is made from cow's milk and sold in small squares, usually in plastic tubs covered in plastic wrap. You can find it in the gourmet or specialty cheese section of your local grocery.

One of the best things about feta is its strong flavor. A little can go a long way. So if you're looking for flavor but don't want to weigh down your food with lots of cheese and fat, feta's a good choice. Look for flavored feta cheese for a change of pace. You can find it blended with sun-dried tomatoes and basil, and peppercorns.

Greek Omelet

Prep time: 5 min • **Cook time:** 10 min • **Yield:** 2 servings

Ingredients	*Directions*
Nonstick cooking spray ½ cup diced green bell peppers ½ cup sliced mushrooms ⅛ teaspoon dried marjoram, crumbled 1 cup chopped spinach 2 whole eggs 4 egg whites ½ cup crumbled feta cheese 1 small plum tomato, seeded and chopped	*1* Coat a large skillet with the cooking spray and place over medium heat. Sauté the peppers, mushrooms, and marjoram until the vegetables are tender, approximately 6 minutes. Add the spinach and cook until wilted, roughly 4 minutes. *2* In a bowl mix together the eggs and egg whites. Pour the egg mixture over the spinach mixture in the skillet. Cook over low heat, stirring occasionally until the eggs are almost cooked. Top with the feta cheese and tomatoes and cover until the eggs are puffy, approximately 5 minutes. Fold the omelet in half and serve.

Per serving: Kcalories 230 (From Fat 120); Fat 13g (Saturated 7g); Cholesterol 246mg; Sodium 607mg; Carbohydrate 8g (Dietary Fiber 2g); Protein 20g.

Vegetable Frittata

Prep time: 25 min • **Cook time:** 15 min • **Yield:** 4 servings

Ingredients	*Directions*
1 pound broccoli	**1** Bring a medium-sized pot of water to the boil. Cut the florets of the broccoli into ½-inch pieces; save the stems for another use like soup. When the water is boiling, sprinkle with salt. Add the broccoli florets. Cook rapidly for about 6 minutes, until the broccoli is tender when pierced with a fork. Drain the broccoli in a colander and let cool. Set aside.
8 eggs	
6 egg whites	
1 tablespoon cold water	
1 pound spinach	
1 tablespoon olive oil	**2** In a mixing bowl, combine eggs, egg whites, and water. Blend thoroughly. Set aside.
2 large onions	
1 large clove garlic	**3** Meanwhile, in a 12-inch oven-safe non-stick sauté pan, cook the onions in the olive oil until soft (3 to 5 minutes). Add the garlic and cook another minute. Add the spinach and cook until wilted. Spread the broccoli over the onion and spinach mixture in the sauté pan. Sprinkle with salt and pepper. Mix together ricotta and white cheese, and spread over broccoli. Pour egg mixture over the broccoli.
½ teaspoon coarse salt	
¼ teaspoon freshly ground black pepper	
¼ cup nonfat ricotta cheese	
¼ cup soft white cheese, such as goat cheese	
¼ cup freshly grated Parmesan cheese	**4** Preheat the broiler.
	5 With a rubber spatula, gently move the vegetables around, making sure the egg goes throughout the broccoli mixture on the bottom of the pan. Don't stir the mixture, but gently move the vegetables, allowing the liquid eggs to reach the surface of the pan. Let the mixture cook over medium-high heat so that a crust forms on the bottom of the pan. With a fork, lift the edges of the frittata and tilt the pan to let the runny eggs go underneath.
	6 When the whole mixture is set, top with the Parmesan cheese and place under the broiler briefly, likely 3 minutes or so, until the top is golden. Serve in wedges for lunch or supper or cut into squares for hors d'oeuvres.

Per serving: Kcalories 377 (Calories from Fat 162); Fat 18g (Saturated 6g); Cholesterol 438mg; Sodium 784mg; Carbohydrate 22g (Dietary Fiber 6.5g); Protein 28g.

Omelet with Wild Mushrooms

Prep time: 25 min • **Cook time:** 15 min • **Yield:** 4 servings

Ingredients	Directions
8 eggs	**1** Crack the eggs and add egg whites into a bowl. Add water, and beat with a fork until the mixture is one color. Set aside.
4 egg whites	
3 tablespoons cold water	
1 tablespoon olive oil, divided	**2** Heat ½ tablespoon olive oil in a small sauté pan, over medium-high heat. Cook the shallots until soft. Add the mushrooms all at once and cook, stirring, until the mushrooms are half wilted. Add the herbs and ricotta cheese. Season to taste with salt and pepper. Continue cooking until the cheese has melted. Remove from the heat.
4 medium shallots, minced	
8 ounces wild or domestic mushrooms, brushed of dirt and cut in ¼-inch slices or pieces	
¼ cup fresh chives, minced	**3** In a medium nonstick sauté pan, heat the remaining ½ tablespoon olive oil over medium-high heat. Pour in the egg mixture, and with a rubber spatula, draw the egg mixture across the pan in one direction and then in the other. You should have a mound of fluffy eggs in the middle of the pan. Let the remaining egg mixture sit and cook for 30 seconds; then, with the rubber spatula, lift the edges of the omelet, and swirl the sauté pan around, to allow the remaining uncooked egg mixture to slide underneath and come into contact with the pan. When all the eggs are lightly cooked, remove the pan from the heat.
¼ cup fresh thyme, minced	
Coarse salt, to taste	
Freshly ground black pepper, to taste	
¼ cup nonfat ricotta cheese	
	4 Cover one half of the open omelet with the mushroom mixture. Then fold over the other half of the omelet. Slide the omelet onto a heated serving plate.

Per serving: Kcalories 240 (Calories from Fat 123); Fat 14g (Saturated 4g); Cholesterol 428mg; Sodium 375mg; Carbohydrate 9g (Dietary Fiber 1g); Protein 20g.

Artichoke Frittata

Prep time: 25 min • **Cook time:** 15 min • **Yield:** 6 servings

Ingredients	Directions
5 large whole frozen artichoke hearts, thawed	*1* Slice the artichoke hearts into ½-inch pieces.
2 teaspoons extra-virgin olive oil **½ teaspoon plus a few pinches salt** **5 eggs** **7 egg whites**	*2* Heat a sauté pan over high heat. Lightly coat the bottom with the olive oil. When the oil begins to shimmer, add the artichoke slices, reduce the heat to medium-low, and sauté the artichokes until they're tender, about 10 minutes, stirring occasionally. Season the artichokes with salt as you sauté them. Remove them from the heat.
1 tablespoon unsalted butter **2 tablespoons finely chopped parsley**	*3* Crack the eggs into a medium bowl. Add the egg whites and season them with a few pinches of salt. Whisk them until they're well blended.
2 tablespoons finely chopped thyme	*4* For a large frittata, heat a large nonstick pan over medium-high heat and then add ½ tablespoon of butter and allow it to coat the bottom of the pan. Place half of the cooked artichoke slices in the pan and sprinkle them with parsley and thyme. Reduce the heat to low and pour half of the egg mixture over the artichokes. Quickly stir everything together so that the artichokes are evenly distributed. Cook the mixture, without stirring, until the eggs are almost set, approximately 4 minutes, and then flip the frittata over and let it cook for another minute or so. Slide out of the pan and onto a serving plate.
	5 Repeat Step 4 to make a second frittata. Cut each frittata into 3 pieces. Serve hot or cold with bread.

Per serving: Kcalories 119 (From Fat 68); Fat 8g (Saturated 3g); Cholesterol 182mg; Sodium 382mg; Carbohydrate 2g (Dietary Fiber 1g); Protein 10g.

Chapter 7

Hors d'Oeuvres and First Courses: Off to a Good Start

In This Chapter

▶ Starting your meal off right

▶ Sampling salsas for every occasion

▶ Digging into delectable dips

Appetizers are meant to stimulate your appetite and prepare you for the meal to come. But for a diabetic, they can also help you squeeze in a quick nutritious bite, helping to keep your blood glucose levels stable until the main event. Healthy appetizers are the best way to get you started on a great eating path for the evening.

In this chapter, we give you many great choices for healthy eats, whether you're having a party, an intimate dinner with friends, or a casual game night with the family. Look here for enticing new ways to enjoy simple finger foods as a first course, terrific salsa recipes with tips for creating your own varieties, and a great selection of dips and dippers — no need to skimp on taste. Just remember to choose appropriate portion sizes and pace yourself. You have a whole lot to enjoy.

Enjoying Simple Starters

Casual dining is definitely on the rise. Many social gatherings focus on food, but may not include a traditional sit-down meal. Instead many people entertain friends and family with "heavy appetizers." We've collected some recipes that are heavy in satisfaction, but won't weigh you down or blow your whole calorie budget for the day.

If your experience with seafood until now has been fish sticks or broiled halibut, we've got some great ideas for getting you going with seafood appetizers. You can experiment with new flavors without committing yourself to a full seafood entree. But be sure to take a look at Chapter 12 for more taste-tempting seafood recipes.

Most people don't get enough seafood in their diet. Rich in fish oil, omega-3 fatty acids, protein, calcium, and so many other nutrients, seafood is an excellent part of any well-rounded diet. This delectable food is much lower in cholesterol than beef and chicken and has so many varied flavors and textures that you can't get bored with it.

Shellfish, such as scallops and shrimp, are sold by weight and size. When you see shrimp labeled as "26/30," you get between 26 and 30 shrimp per pound. So the higher the number, the smaller the shrimp, and vice versa. You may even see labels that say "U10," which means "under 10," or fewer than 10 shrimp per pound.

Always clean your shrimp properly before cooking them. If you buy your shrimp in a grocery store, the head will most likely be removed. But the shrimp may or may not be deveined, which means the dark "vein" that runs down the back of the shrimp's tail may still be present. Because this veinlike object is actually the shrimp's intestinal track, you should remove it before cooking the shrimp. At your grocery or kitchen supply store (anywhere kitchen gadgets are sold), pick up a tool called a shrimp deveiner and run it along the back end of the shrimp. It cracks the shell and removes the vein in one easy step. Then rinse the shrimp in cool water. Check out Figure 7-1 to see the deveining process.

Figure 7-1:
You can use a special tool to clean and devein shrimp safely and properly.

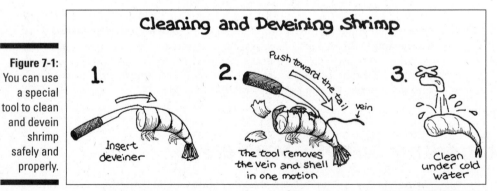

Cleaning and Deveining Shrimp

1. Insert deveiner

2. Push toward the tail — vein. The tool removes the vein and shell in one motion

3. Clean under cold water

Illustration by Elizabeth Kurtzman

Shrimp Quesadillas

Prep time: 15 min • **Cook time:** 10 min • **Yield:** 4 servings

Ingredients	Directions
⅓ cup lowfat sugar-free plain yogurt	*1* In a small bowl, combine the yogurt and tomatoes. Set aside.
2 medium plum tomatoes, seeded and chopped	
Nonstick cooking spray	*2* Coat a large skillet with the cooking spray. Place the skillet over medium heat until hot. Add one tortilla to the pan. Top the tortilla with half of the shrimp, 1 teaspoon of the chopped cilantro, and ½ cup of cheese. Place a second tortilla on top of the mixture. Cook the quesadilla until the cheese begins to melt and the bottom tortilla becomes golden brown. Flip the quesadilla over and continue to cook until the cheese is fully melted and the tortillas are lightly browned. Remove from skillet and place on a cutting board.
4 10-inch whole-wheat tortillas	
1 pound canned baby shrimp, cooked	
2 teaspoons fresh cilantro, chopped	
1 cup (4 ounces) shredded Monterey Jack cheese	*3* Repeat Step 2 with the remaining tortillas, shrimp, cilantro, and cheese.
	4 Slice each quesadilla into 6 pieces. Place 3 pieces and one-fourth of the tomato mixture on each of 4 plates.

Per serving: Kcalories 364 (From Fat 112); Fat 13g (Saturated 6g); Cholesterol 204mg; Sodium 1,653mg; Carbohydrate 33g (Dietary Fiber 6g); Protein 29g.

Pickled Sardine Appetizer

Prep time: 1 hr • **Cool time:** 3 hr • **Cook time:** 7 min • **Yield:** 6 servings

Ingredients	Directions
½ cup salt 2 quarts water	**1** In a medium bowl, add the ½ cup salt to the water and dissolve the salt.
2 pounds fresh rinsed sardine filet 2 teaspoons yellow mustard seed	**2** In a large baking dish, place the sardine filet. Pour the saltwater over the sardines. Allow the sardines to brine for 12 hours. The sardine brine is good up to 2 weeks.
2 teaspoons allspice berry 4 teaspoons peppercorn 6 bay leaves 6 cloves	**3** Heat a heavy skillet over medium heat until hot. Add the mustard seed, allspice berry, 4 teaspoons peppercorn, bay leaves, and cloves; toast 2 to 5 minutes or until spices are fragrant and lightly browned, stirring constantly to prevent burning. Remove from heat. Combine in a cheesecloth.
½ cup sugar 1 quart white wine vinegar 2 Meyer lemons, slivered in rings	**4** In a medium saucepan, bring the sugar and white wine vinegar to a boil until dissolved. Remove from the heat and add the slivered lemons and onion. Set aside to cool.
1 red onion 2 teaspoons fennel 2 teaspoons coriander	**5** Discard the solids and pour this liquid over the sardines. It will be ready to use in 3 hours and will keep for up to 3 weeks.
1 teaspoon pink peppercorn ½ teaspoon salt	**6** Toast the 2 teaspoons fennel, coriander, pink peppercorn, and ½ teaspoon salt. Crush roughly in a mortar.
¼ cup orange juice concentrate ⅓ cup golden balsamic vinegar ½ cup extra-virgin olive oil	**7** In a large bowl, combine the orange juice concentrate, balsamic vinegar, ½ cup extra-virgin olive oil, and salt to taste.

Salt to taste

2 green heart radish or turnip, sliced thinly on a mandolin

8 kumquats, sliced thinly on a mandolin

2 oranges, sliced to ¼-inch thickness

1 medium bulb fennel, shaved thinly

1 bunch parsley, leaves only

½ Serrano, seeded

¼ cup extra-virgin olive oil (just enough to blend)

1 clove roasted garlic or 2 teaspoons raw garlic

1 Meyer lemon, zested

2 teaspoons lemon juice

8 Toss the radish or turnip, kumquats, oranges, fennel bulb, and the red onion from Step 4 in the large bowl from Step 7. Arrange the mixture on a plate and sprinkle with the toasted seed mixture from Step 6.

9 In a blender, puree the parsley, Serrano, ¼ cup extra-virgin olive oil, roasted garlic, zested lemon, and lemon juice to make a pesto. Dot the plate in Step 8 with the pesto.

Per serving: Kcalories 403 (From Fat 342); Fat 38g (Saturated Fat 3g); Cholesterol 214mg; Sodium 7mg; Carbohydrate 15g (Dietary Fiber 3g); Protein 1g.

Crab Puffs

Prep time: 20 min • **Cook time:** 6–7 min • **Yield:** 6 servings (4 pieces each)

Ingredients	Directions
3 tablespoons freshly grated Parmesan cheese	*1* Preheat the broiler.
1 can (14 ounces) artichoke hearts, drained and chopped	*2* In a small bowl, reserve 2 tablespoons of the Parmesan cheese. In a medium bowl, combine the remaining 1 tablespoon Parmesan cheese, the chopped artichokes, crabmeat, egg white, sour cream, mayonnaise, lemon juice, horseradish, Worcestershire sauce, and garlic.
½ pound snow crabmeat	
1 egg white	
¼ cup lowfat sour cream	
¼ cup lowfat mayonnaise	*3* Place the English muffin halves on a baking pan and spread the crab mixture equally onto each muffin. Sprinkle the reserved Parmesan cheese on top.
1 teaspoon fresh squeezed lemon juice	
1 teaspoon prepared horseradish	*4* Place the pan in the freezer for 10 minutes, or until the crab mixture holds its form.
½ teaspoon Worcestershire sauce	*5* Remove the pan from the freezer and place the pan under the broiler for 6 to 7 minutes, or until the muffin topping is lightly browned and bubbly. Cut each muffin into quarters.
1 small garlic clove, minced	
3 English muffins, halved	

Per serving: Kcalories 180 (From Fat 47); Fat 5g (Saturated 2g); Cholesterol 41mg; Sodium 536mg; Carbohydrate 20g (Dietary Fiber 1g); Protein 13g.

Vary It! If you're a fan of spicy food, feel free to bump up the horseradish in this recipe for a sinus-clearing experience.

Savoring Salsas

We've fallen in love with the Mexican condiment, salsa. Most store-bought versions, however, have too much sugar and vinegar, so they aren't nearly as good as the homemade variety. Why bother with those versions when it's so easy to create your own? Although *salsa* simply means "sauce," we think you'll agree that these salsa recipes taste anything but simple.

Stocking essentials for scrumptious salsas

Add the standard salsa seasonings to any grain or legume for a tasty and nutritious treat anytime. You can flavor cooked brown rice, quinoa, or any cooked beans with any of these tasty additions:

- ✔ Cilantro
- ✔ Garlic
- ✔ Lime juice or lemon juice
- ✔ Onions
- ✔ Peppers (such as serranos and jalapeños)
- ✔ Tomatoes

Check out the following salsa recipes, which use these delicious ingredients.

Use caution when slicing and dicing hot peppers such as jalapeños. Use your knife, not your fingers or fingernails, to remove the super-spicy ribs and seeds, and consider wearing gloves if you have sensitive skin. The pepper oil can get stuck under your nails, making it painful to touch your eyes, nose, or any other moist parts later. And if your skin is exposed to sunlight with residual pepper oil, you can get a nasty burn.

Mexican Salsa

Prep time: 10 min • **Yield:** 4 servings

Ingredients	Directions
½ teaspoon lemon juice ½ teaspoon salt	**1** In a mixing bowl, combine the lemon juice and salt. Stir to dissolve the salt.
1 pound fresh tomatoes, cored and chopped ½ medium onion, diced 1 tablespoon fresh chopped jalapeño pepper 1 small garlic clove, chopped fine 1 teaspoon fresh chopped cilantro	**2** Add the tomatoes and coat them with the juice. Add the onion, jalapeño, garlic, and cilantro and stir.

Per serving: Kcalories 30 (From Fat 4); Fat 0g (Saturated 0g); Cholesterol 0mg; Sodium 301mg; Carbohydrate 7g (Dietary Fiber 2g); Protein 1g.

Tip: If you like a smooth rather than chunky salsa, toss all the ingredients in a food processor and process the mixture in pulses until it reaches the consistency you desire.

Adding citrus and other fruits to salsas

To give your salsa a fruity twist, don't bother with bottled lemon or lime juice. Fresh is definitely the way to go. Squeezing the juice out is easy to do, and the flavor is far superior.

Here's how to get the most out of your citrus fruit. Check out Figure 7-2 for details.

1. **Roll the fruit on a hard, flat surface, pressing down fairly hard to break up the juice sacs.**

2. **Cut the citrus fruit in half width-wise.**

3. **Holding one half in one hand, stick the tines of a fork into the fruit pulp and squeeze the fruit.**

   Twist the fork as needed to release as much juice as possible.

Juice your fruit over a separate bowl, not into other ingredients. Doing so helps you catch any errant seeds that may try to sneak their way into your delectable dishes.

Lemon and lime aren't the only fruity flavors you can add to your salsas. Check out the following yummy salsas featuring mango and pineapple.

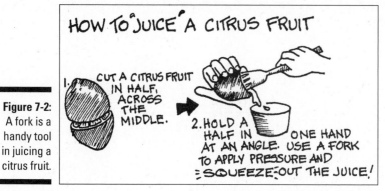

Figure 7-2:
A fork is a handy tool in juicing a citrus fruit.

Illustration by Elizabeth Kurtzman

Mango Salsa

Prep time: 15 min • **Yield:** 4 servings

Ingredients	Directions
1 large ripe mango, peeled, pitted, and chopped	In a mixing bowl, combine all the ingredients and mix well. Cover and refrigerate until ready to serve.
½ small red bell pepper, seeded and chopped	
1 medium tomato, seeded and cubed	
1 green onion, green and white parts, chopped	
2 tablespoons minced fresh ginger	
Juice of 1 lime	
3 tablespoons fresh chopped cilantro	

Per serving: Kcalories 50 (From Fat 3); Fat 0g (Saturated 0g); Cholesterol 0mg; Sodium 4mg; Carbohydrate 13g (Dietary Fiber 2g); Protein 1g.

Warm Pineapple Salsa

Prep time: 20 min • **Cook time:** 15 min • **Yield:** 4 servings

Ingredients	Directions
1 tablespoon olive oil	**1** In a small saucepan, heat the oil over medium heat. Add the almonds and gently toss in the oil.
1 tablespoon slivered almonds	
1 small onion, thinly sliced	**2** Add the onion and cook until tender and until the almonds are golden brown.
2 teaspoons curry powder	
16 ounces pineapple tidbits, drained	**3** Add the curry powder, pineapple, vinegar, salt, honey, and raisins. Bring the mixture to a boil, reduce the heat, and simmer for 10 minutes. Remove the salsa from the heat and serve warm.
1 tablespoon cider vinegar	
¼ teaspoon salt	
1 tablespoon honey	
1 tablespoon brown seedless raisins	

Vary It! Try this recipe with canned mandarin oranges, apricots, or peaches instead of the pineapple, depending on your accompaniments and your taste buds on a given day. But be sure to avoid fruit packed in heavy syrup.

Per serving: Kcalories 114 (From Fat 40); Fat 5g (Saturated 1g); Cholesterol 0mg; Sodium 148mg; Carbohydrate 20g (Dietary Fiber 1g); Protein 1g.

Discovering Delicious Dips

Dips don't have to be fat-laden creamy concoctions that add inches to your waistline and bags to your saddle. With a little creativity, you can create delicious dips that keep you eating healthy and your glucose levels normal.

Whipping up dips with pantry staples

Dips are among the quickest and easiest (not to mention tastiest!) appetizers around. Keep your pantry and fridge stocked with a few dip-making essentials and you'll never be stuck wondering what to whip up when unexpected guests stop by.

Here are our best bets for quick dip-making essentials to keep on hand:

- ✔ **Any of the ingredients listed under "Stocking essentials for scrumptious salsas," earlier in this chapter:** Adding any of the salsa ingredients to any of the items in this list makes for a terrific dip. In fact, one of our favorite quick dips blends a can of black beans (rinsed and drained, of course) with ½ cup of salsa. Whip the mixture in a food processor, and you have an instant party treat.

- ✔ **Beans:** Pureed beans make a great base for a dip, and they're high in fiber and low in fat. Blend them in a food processor and season them with your favorite spices. Look for fat-free, low-sodium canned beans, and try cannellini beans, black beans, pinto beans, black-eyed peas, garbanzo beans, great Northern beans, navy beans, and kidney beans.

  Unless a recipe says otherwise, rinse and drain canned beans before adding them to a dip. Often, the liquid they're canned in is salty or flavored in some way. Rinse and drain and season them your way.

- ✔ **Fancy olives:** Olives impart great flavor and texture to dips. Use some of the olive juice to blend into the dip, too. If olives perk up a martini, just think what they can do for some ho-hum dips!

- ✔ **Fresh herbs:** Fresh herbs make an instant impression on an otherwise bland dip base. Dill, basil, and cilantro are excellent choices for keeping on hand.

- ✔ **Lowfat sour cream:** Use sour cream to add a little body and creamy texture to your dips.

- ✔ **Plain yogurt:** This staple is a natural partner to fresh herbs and a touch of lemon juice. Keep it handy to mix in a soon-to-be bean dip.

- ✔ **Spice blends:** Look for prepackaged, salt-free spice blends. These healthy spices can take the guesswork out of seasoning.

White Bean Dip

Prep time: 10 min • **Chill time:** 3–4 hr • **Cook time:** 5 min • **Yield:** 4 servings

Ingredients	Directions
Nonstick cooking spray ½ cup chopped onions 2 garlic cloves, minced	*1* Place a medium skillet over medium heat and coat it with nonstick cooking spray. Add the onions and cook until they're soft and translucent, about 1 minute.
1 can (15 ounces) cannellini beans, drained and rinsed	*2* Add the garlic and continue to cook for about 30 seconds.
½ teaspoon chopped fresh sage 1 teaspoon balsamic vinegar 1 tablespoon water	*3* Place the beans in a food processor and add the cooked onions and garlic, sage, vinegar, water, salt, and pepper. Process until smooth (about 1 to 2 minutes).
⅛ teaspoon salt ⅛ teaspoon pepper	*4* Transfer the mixture to a bowl, cover it, and refrigerate it for 3 to 4 hours before serving.

Per serving: Kcalories 65 (From Fat 3); Fat 0g (Saturated 1g); Cholesterol 0mg; Sodium 161mg; Carbohydrate 12g (Dietary Fiber 3g); Protein 3g.

Cacit (Cucumber Dip)

Prep time: 10 min • **Stand time:** 2 hr • **Yield:** 4 servings

Ingredients	*Directions*
1 English cucumber (or 4 small)	**1** Cut the cucumber into 1-inch dices. Place the cucumber in a stainless steel colander, and sprinkle with salt. Let the cucumbers drain for 1 to 2 hours, to remove excess liquid.
2 garlic cloves	
½ teaspoon coarse salt	
2 tablespoons minced fresh mint	**2** On a cutting board, make a paste of the garlic with the salt. Place garlic mixture in a bowl. Add the cucumbers, mint, and yogurt. Mix well and add salt to taste.
1 cup nonfat Greek-style yogurt	

Per serving: Calories 40 (From Fat 0); Fat 0g (Saturated 0g); Cholesterol 0mg; Sodium 313mg; Carbohydrate 4g; Dietary Fiber 1g; Protein 6g.

Tuna Pâté

Prep time: 10 min • **Chill time:** 3–4 hr • **Yield:** 6 servings

Ingredients	Directions
½ small onion	**1** In a food processor, combine the onion, cilantro, and jalapeño and pulse until chopped, approximately 1 minute.
2 teaspoons fresh cilantro	
1 tablespoon chopped jalapeño pepper	
12 ounces canned tuna, packed in water, drained	**2** Add the tuna and process approximately 1 minute.
½ cup mayonnaise	**3** Slowly add the mayonnaise and process until smooth, approximately 30 seconds.
⅛ teaspoon white pepper	**4** Add the pepper and process 1 minute. Check for lumps and process until smooth. Transfer the dip to a serving bowl, chill it for 3 to 4 hours, and serve.

Per serving: Kcalories 195 (From Fat 144); Fat 16g (Saturated 3g); Cholesterol 30mg; Sodium 283mg; Carbohydrate 1g (Dietary Fiber 0g); Protein 11g.

Choosing healthy dippers

What's a good dip without something to dip into it? Rather than ruining all your hard work of choosing healthy dips by dipping fried chips into them, we offer you the following alternatives to keep you moving in the right direction:

- **Bagel chips:** Look for these chips in the specialty bread section of your grocery store, but read the label because some are high in fat and sodium. You also can make your own by slicing off slivers of a bagel and then baking them until they're crisp.

- **Fresh veggies:** Choose broccoli florets, cauliflower florets, carrot sticks, celery sticks, zucchini slices, red pepper spears, endive scoops, or any of your favorites. Any veggie can be a dip delivery system.

- **Pita wedges:** Make your own by quartering pitas and then baking them until they're crisp.

- **Whole-wheat crackers:** Kashi makes a line called TLC, Tasty Little Crackers, made with whole-grain flour from seven different grains. Ry-Krisp is a filling and tasty choice as well.

- **Yucca chips:** This root vegetable has great health benefits. Check out the following recipe.

Yucca Chips

Prep time: 10 min • **Cook time:** 45 min • **Yield:** 4 servings

Ingredients	*Directions*
⅛ **teaspoon salt**	*1* Preheat the oven to 375 degrees.
⅛ **teaspoon pepper**	
2 large yucca, peeled and cut into wedges	*2* In a small bowl, combine the salt and pepper. In a large bowl, coat the yucca wedges with the olive oil and then toss them with the salt and pepper.
2 tablespoons extra-virgin olive oil	
Nonstick cooking spray	*3* Coat a baking sheet with cooking spray and arrange the wedges on the sheet. Bake about 45 minutes, or until the yucca wedges are cooked through and lightly browned.

Per serving: Kcalories 386 (From Fat 66); Fat 7g (Saturated 1g); Cholesterol 0mg; Sodium 101mg; Carbohydrate 78g (Dietary Fiber 4g); Protein 3g.

Chapter 8

The Benefits of Soup

Soups might be the ultimate comfort food. Who doesn't feel better (even with a cold) with a bowl of warm chicken soup? And you can choose a soup for every occasion. No matter what the weather, the state of your health, or who's coming for dinner, we have a soup for you.

In this chapter, we get you started with the basics of making soup, taking you through the steps to make sure your soups turn out just right. We give you the scoop on different types of stocks, provide tips on watching your salt intake, and help you get your pantry stocked for soup making. We give you tips on making healthful, creamy soups full of flavor, but low in fat. And finally, we help you make delicious soups to serve cold on warm summer days.

Understanding Soup-Making Basics

In many soup recipes, the first few steps ask you to sauté some vegetables to bring out their flavor and soften them. Typically, you start by cooking a combination of vegetables, such as onions, carrots, and celery, along with herbs and spices, in a small amount of fat.

You may sauté your veggies in a small amount of lowfat cooking spray oil or butter, or even a bit of fatty smoked meat such as bacon. You may also brown ground meats or cubed meats at this stage. As the ingredients cook, they begin to turn brown and *caramelize,* developing a rich and complex flavor.

Next, you add liquid, perhaps some vegetable broth, chicken or beef broth, milk, wine, or water. First, add just a half-cup or so of liquid to *deglaze* the pot. During this procedure, you can use a wooden spoon and gently dislodge any bits of caramelized vegetables stuck to the bottom of the pot. You want these flavorful morsels to blend in with the other flavors of the soup. Pour in the remaining liquid.

In the final, and longest, steps of cooking, you place all vegetable chunks, beans, grains, or meats, in the simmering liquid and cook to perfection. But not everything cooks at the same rate, so use Table 8-1 to help you decide when to add ingredients.

Table 8-1	Cooking Times for Soup Add-Ins
Ingredient	*Cooking Time*
Beans, dried (presoaked 8 hours)	1½ hours to 2 hours
Beef cubes	2 to 3 hours
Chicken, bone in, pieces	40 minutes
Chicken, boneless	15 to 20 minutes
Fresh vegetables	10 to 15 minutes (45 to purée)
Greens (spinach and others)	3 to 5 minutes
Lentils, dried	15 to 30 minutes
Pasta, dried	8 to 12 minutes
Pearl barley	50 minutes to 1 hour
Potatoes, white or sweet (diced)	30 minutes
Rice, brown and wild	45 to 55 minutes
Rice, white	15 to 20 minutes
Root vegetables (beets, turnips, and so on)	15 to 35 minutes
Seafood, shelled or boneless	5 to 15 minutes

These cooking times are only guidelines, so adjust them as you see fit. Experiment and figure out what works for you.

Soups are a great way to work in your veggies. Use soups as a way to maximize the bounty of summer vegetables at your local farmer's market, especially at the end of the season. Look for these must-have ingredients that have a place in soups, salads, or even quick-cooking pasta sauces:

✔ Beets

✔ Greens (spinach, cabbage, and bok choy, among others)

✔ Heirloom tomatoes (look for green zebras, Japanese black trifle, sun sugar, or amana orange, just to name a few)

✔ Herbs (basil, chervil, dill, and cilantro, or whatever you want)

✔ Mushrooms (exotics, such as morels, chanterelle, and wild mushroom blends)

✔ Squash (chayote, acorn, pumpkin, zucchini, and yellow squash)

Stock up on heirloom tomatoes to make the next quick and tasty recipe.

Heirloom Tomato Soup with Fresh Basil

Prep time: 20 min • **Cook time:** 30 min • **Yield:** 4 servings

Ingredients	Directions
2 tablespoons extra-virgin olive oil	**1** Heat olive oil in a heavy bottomed skillet over medium heat. Stir in the garlic and let cook gently until it turns slightly golden — be careful not to let the garlic burn.
5 large fresh heirloom tomatoes, peeled, seeded, and chopped into ½-inch dice	
5 garlic cloves, peeled and minced	**2** Immediately stir in the tomatoes and gently sauté until slightly thickened, about 5 minutes. Stir in the stock and let simmer another 10 to 15 minutes. Stir in the basil and let the soup simmer gently 2 or 3 minutes more.
1 quart good quality low-sodium or vegetable stock, heated	
1 teaspoon coarse salt	**3** Serve soup in warmed bowls. Top with Parmesan cheese.
Freshly ground black pepper	
30 fresh basil leaves, thinly sliced	
¼ cup freshly grated Parmesan cheese	

Note: The best way to peel and seed tomatoes is to blanch and shock them, to loosen the skin. Start by removing the stem end of the tomato with a small knife. Make an "x" in the opposite end of the tomato with the knife. Drop the tomatoes in gently boiling water for no longer than 10 seconds. Immediately transfer them to a bowl of cold water. Then gently peel off the loosened skins. To seed them, cut the tomatoes in half with the stem end on one side. Over fine mesh strainer fitted onto a bowl or measuring cup, use one hand to scoop out the seeds, while squeezing the tomato half with the other. Don't worry if you don't get out all the seeds. A couple of seeds won't hurt anyone.

Per serving: Kcalories 167 (Calories from Fat 86); Fat 10g (Saturated 2g); Cholesterol 4mg; Sodium 1,155mg; Carbohydrate 17g (Dietary Fiber 4g); Protein 5g.

Serving Up Soups with Stocks and Other Essentials

You can begin a soup using water, but making a soup with real depth of flavor calls for stock. Basically, a *stock* is a liquid in which solid ingredients, such as chicken meat and bones, vegetables, and spices, are cooked and then usually strained out. The flavors of these ingredients end up in the final broth.

Look for *stock bases,* the secret ingredient of many a restaurant, near the bouillon and broth in your grocery store. Usually sold in one-pound containers, you can make up to five gallons of stock from a single container. Keeping a container of base in the fridge is more convenient than keeping five gallons of canned broth in your pantry.

Watching out for salt in stock-based soups

Most markets carry various brands of chicken and beef broth that offer good flavor. These products are adequate for making everyday soups and are well worth keeping on hand. Always choose the low-sodium versions to use as stock and then add more salt to your soup as necessary.

If your physician or dietitian has given you any instructions at all about watching your salt, you've probably been told about the high sodium content of canned soup. You may be on a standard 3,000-milligrams-a-day regimen, recommended for most individuals, or a 2,000-milligrams-a-day sodium-restricted diet. Table 8-2 shows some sample amounts of the milligrams of sodium in a single serving of some common soups.

Table 8-2	Canned Soups and Sodium	
Soups	*Serving Size*	*Sodium in Milligrams*
Low Sodium Tomato (Campbell's)	10½ ounces	60
Low Sodium Chicken Broth (Campbell's)	10½ ounces	140
Chicken Broth (Health Valley)	8 ounces	150
Onion Soup Mix (Lipton)	8 ounces (or 1 tablespoon mix)	610
Lentil (Progresso)	8 ounces	750
Tomato (Campbell's)	4 ounces (condensed soup)	760

(continued)

Table 8-2 *(continued)*

Soups	Serving Size	Sodium in Milligrams
Chicken Broth (Campbell's)	4 ounces (condensed soup)	770
Vegetable Beef (Campbell's)	4 ounces (condensed soup)	890
Chicken Noodle Instant Soup (Knorr)	8 ounces	910
Clam Chowder (Campbell's)	4 ounces (condensed soup)	960
Chunky Beef (Campbell's)	10¾ ounces	1,130

For another low-salt stock alternative, you can make a basic vegetable stock by simmering together aromatic vegetables like onion and celery with carrots, which add sweetness, plus some parsley and a bay leaf. You need to cook this mixture for only about 20 minutes.

The classical combination of vegetables (onions, celery, and carrots) is called *mirepoix* (pronounced *meer*-pwa). It's a basic beginning for many soups and stocks. When you're chopping mirepoix for stocks, you can roughly chop the vegetables and even skip the peeling if you prefer. But when getting the veggies ready for soups, take the time to prep them as the recipe suggests.

Keeping soup supplies in your pantry

Different types of stocks aren't the only items you need to have close by when you're craving soup. Keep the following ingredients in your pantry for an impromptu soup-making session:

✔ **Canned evaporated milk:** Use this item in your creamy soup recipes. Evaporated milk is *not* the same as sweetened condensed milk (a syrupy milk-based concoction with lots of sugar added). Evaporated milk is milk from which 60 percent of the water has been removed. It's concentrated, so it can enhance the flavor of soups and other dishes.

Choose regular evaporated milk rather than evaporated skim milk for soups and sauces. Evaporated skim milk has a tendency to curdle and break when heated. If you still want to save the calories, purée the soup with the skim milk before serving.

✔ **Canned legumes, like beans, lentils, and chickpeas:** They're a great source of fiber and protein, but the dried variety can take some time to prepare. So have the canned variety available to toss in a soup pot in a pinch. Get started using these hearty staples in the Indian-Inspired Lamb and Legume Chili later in this chapter.

Always drain and rinse canned beans and vegetables unless the recipe specifies otherwise. This step removes excess sodium, allowing you to season your soup to your preferred taste.

✔ **Canned tomatoes:** Diced, crushed, whole, or stewed, any of these tomatoes products can make for a quick soup.

✔ **Dried herbs and spices:** Oregano, basil, pepper, salt, dill, and just about anything in your spice cabinet can work into a soup recipe.

✔ **Dried mushrooms:** Rehydrate them in hot water, steep them for about 30 minutes, and then strain the liquid to remove any grit. Roughly chop the mushrooms and add the strained liquid for an extra punch of flavor.

✔ **Garlic:** Garlic adds an amazing flavor to just about anything. You can roast it, sauté it, and purée it; whatever works for your soup. It's great in creamy soups, tomato-based soups, or brothy soups. (Not intended for any visiting vampires eating soup, and don't forget the breath mints.)

✔ **Grains:** Rice, pasta, and barley are great choices to make a soup heartier. Check out Chapter 10 for the full story on cooking with grains.

✔ **Olive oil:** This terrific monounsaturated fat can help make an already nutritious soup heart healthy, too. Keep some on hand at all times.

✔ **Onions:** These fragrant bulbs add their terrific flavor and aroma to anything you cook.

✔ **Potatoes:** These starchy veggies cook up quickly and can add body to your soups. Choose them for puréed soups as they help thicken soups almost instantly, like in the Potato-Leek Soup later in this chapter.

✔ **Salt-free seasoning mixes:** If you have trouble with high blood pressure, you probably need to steer clear of salt as much as possible. Salt-free seasoning blends can give you many delicious flavor combinations and take the guesswork out of seasoning your soups.

Potato-Leek Soup

Prep time: 20 min • **Cook time:** 25 min • **Yield:** 4 servings

Ingredients	*Directions*
Nonstick cooking spray	*1* Coat a large pot with cooking spray and place over medium heat until hot. Add the leeks. Sauté until soft and translucent.
1 large leek, chopped and rinsed (don't use the dark green part of leek)	
2 cups potatoes, peeled and cut into ¼-inch cubes	*2* Add the potatoes and chicken broth. Bring to a boil and simmer for 10 to 15 minutes, until the potatoes are cooked. Add the pepper and salt. Continue to simmer for 2 minutes. Remove from the heat.
2 cups low-sodium chicken broth	
¼ teaspoon pepper	*3* Place half of contents of the pot into a blender, cover, and process until smooth.
⅛ teaspoon salt	
	4 Carefully pour the blender mixture back into the pot with the remaining broth and potatoes. Stir together with a wire whisk. Bring back to a simmer.

Per serving: Kcalories 87 (From Fat 8); Fat 1g (Saturated 0g); Cholesterol 2mg; Sodium 134mg; Carbohydrate 17g (Dietary Fiber 2g); Protein 3g.

Tip: Check out Figure 8-1 to see how to cut up a leek. Swish sliced leeks around in a bowl of cold water. Soak them for a few minutes until the dirt and grit settle to the bottom of the bowl. Lift the leeks out of the water and drain on a paper towel. Repeat the procedure again with fresh water.

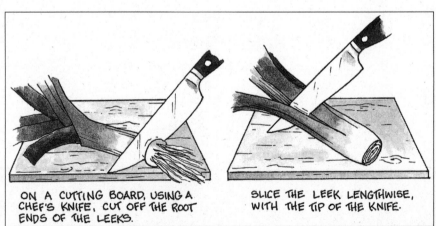

Figure 8-1: Cutting up a leek.

ON A CUTTING BOARD, USING A CHEF'S KNIFE, CUT OFF THE ROOT ENDS OF THE LEEKS.

SLICE THE LEEK LENGTHWISE, WITH THE TIP OF THE KNIFE.

Illustration by Elizabeth Kurtzman

Hearty Vegetable Soup

Prep time: 15 min • **Cook time:** 30 min • **Yield:** 4 servings

Ingredients	Directions
Nonstick cooking spray	**1** Choose a large pot with a tightly fitting lid. Coat the pot with the nonstick spray and cook, stirring constantly, the onions, celery, and carrots until the onions are translucent — about 5 to 7 minutes. You can spray the pot with additional cooking spray or add a little stock or water if the vegetables begin to stick or burn. Add the yucca, tomatoes, zucchini, bay leaf, thyme, oregano, chicken broth, and white pepper and stir to combine.
½ cup diced onions	
½ cup diced celery	
½ cup diced carrots	
1 cup diced fresh yucca	
½ cup diced fresh tomatoes	
½ cup diced zucchini	**2** Bring the vegetable soup to a boil over high heat, uncovered, and then simmer, covered, for 20 minutes.
1 bay leaf	
⅛ teaspoon thyme	**3** Remove the bay leaf and serve immediately as a light lunch or mini meal.
½ teaspoon oregano	
2 cups low-sodium chicken broth	
⅛ teaspoon white pepper	

Per serving: Kcalories 124 (From Fat 10); Fat 1g (Saturated 1g); Cholesterol 2mg; Sodium 85mg; Carbohydrate 26g (Dietary Fiber 3g); Protein 3g.

Note: Adding salt is optional, but it does increase the sodium level.

Lentil Soup with Spinach

Prep time: 10 min • **Cook time:** 35 min • **Yield:** 6 servings

Ingredients	*Directions*
1½ cups red lentils, picked over and rinsed	*1* In a large soup pot, place the lentils.
5 cups water	*2* Add the water, tomatoes, olive oil, garlic cloves, ginger, rosemary, and bay leaf.
One 28-ounce can diced fire-roasted tomatoes	
2 tablespoons extra-virgin olive oil	*3* Increase the heat to high and bring to a boil.
8 cloves garlic, peeled, diced	*4* When the soup starts to boil, reduce the heat to medium or medium-low and allow to simmer until the lentils are soft, about 30 minutes.
5 slices peeled ginger, ⅛-inch thick, diced	
3 sprigs fresh rosemary	
1 bay leaf	*5* Add the salt and pepper. Stir well.
2 teaspoons salt	
Pepper to taste	*6* Add the spinach and lemon juice.
16 ounces baby spinach, rinsed (and chopped, if desired)	
2 tablespoons lemon juice	

Per Serving: Kcalories 223 (From Fat 9); Fat 1g (Saturated Fat 0g); Cholesterol 0mg; Sodium 396mg; Carbohydrate 39g (Dietary Fiber 19g); Protein 15g.

Modifying classic favorites with an international kick

Soups are part of every cuisine. And virtually any soup can get a little ethnic flavor by changing the spices and seasonings (all of which are found in most kitchens). In the next recipe, the garam masala, a traditional Indian spice blend, gives this chili a taste of India. You can find this tasty spice blend in the spice section of most grocery stores now. If you want to change the flavors to match another culture's cuisine, change the seasonings.

Try these few ideas to substitute for the garam masala, changing the flavor, but keeping the basic recipe.

- ✔ Chinese five-spice powder, ground ginger, and a touch of sesame oil stirred in at the end of cooking, for a Chinese-inspired chili

- ✔ Chili powder and cayenne, for a traditional southwestern chili

- ✔ Cinnamon, for a Cincinnati-style chili

- ✔ Basil, marjoram, oregano, thyme, and rosemary, for a taste of Italy

- ✔ Thyme, cinnamon, ginger, allspice, cloves, garlic, and onions, for a little Jamaican jerk flavor

- ✔ Cumin, coriander seed, and cloves, for a taste of North Africa

Indian-Inspired Lamb and Legume Chili

Prep time: 10 min • **Cook time:** 2½ hours (largely unattended) • **Yield:** 8 servings

Ingredients	Directions
1½ pounds lean ground lamb	*1* Combine the lamb, onion, and garlic in a large stockpot. Cook over medium heat until the lamb is browned and crumbled, about 5 minutes. Stir as needed. Drain in a colander to remove excess fat. Return drained meat mixture to the stockpot.
1 cup chopped red onion	
3 garlic cloves, minced	
2 cans (14½ ounces each) no-salt-added diced tomatoes, undrained	
1 cup dry red wine	*2* Stir in the tomatoes, wine, chili powder, coriander, garam masala, and chilies. Bring to a boil. Cover, reduce heat, and cook 2 hours, stirring occasionally.
1 tablespoon chili powder	
1½ teaspoons ground coriander	*3* Stir in the black beans, lentils, and chickpeas. Simmer an additional 30 minutes. Serve immediately.
1½ teaspoons garam masala	
¼ cup serrano chilies, seeded and minced (about 2 chilies)	
1 can (15 ounces) black beans, drained and rinsed	
1 can (15 ounces) lentils, drained and rinsed	
1 can (15 ounces) chickpeas, drained and rinsed	

Per serving: Kcalories 311 (From Fat 126); Fat 14g (Saturated 6g); Cholesterol 61mg; Sodium 248mg; Carbohydrate 23g (Dietary Fiber 9g); Protein 23g.

Tip: Lamb tends to be a high-fat meat, however, so be sure to drain the fat during the cooking process.

Creating Creamy Concoctions

Who doesn't love a delicious creamy soup? But as you probably know, putting cream in soups adds calories *and* saturated fat, neither of which is very good for a diabetic diet. If you can't get enough of creamy soups, we have some good news. You can have a great creamy texture — without the stuff you don't need.

One great way to get the creamy texture without the bad stuff is to substitute 2 percent milk for cream in your favorite soups. It gives you plenty of the creaminess and mouth feel you expect because it does have some fat and body, but it cuts the fat grams and calories.

Top your soup with beautiful garnishes to make a simple weeknight supper as delicious for your eyes as it is to your tummy. A few of our favorite fresh garnishes include the following:

- ✔ Chiffonade basil (see Chapter 9 for an explanation of chiffonade)
- ✔ Diced red bell pepper
- ✔ Finely grated lemon zest
- ✔ Grated or shaved Parmesan cheese and minced parsley
- ✔ Julienned radishes, jicama (see Figure 8-2), or daikon radish
- ✔ A dollop of light sour cream and cilantro
- ✔ Minced olives
- ✔ Thinly sliced green onions

Figure 8-2: Jicama is a crunchy vegetable with a thin brown skin and white flesh.

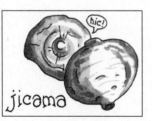

Illustration by Elizabeth Kurtzman

Cauliflower-Parmesan Soup

Prep time: 15 min • **Cook time:** 40–45 min • **Yield:** 4 servings

Ingredients	Directions
1 head cauliflower cut into chunks	**1** In a large pot, place the cauliflower, shallots, and milk and bring to a boil. Reduce heat to a simmer until the cauliflower is tender, about 35 minutes.
2 shallots, chopped	
3 cups 2 percent milk	
½ cup grated Parmesan cheese	**2** Transfer to a blender and purée until smooth (always be extra careful when blending hot liquids), or use a rotary beater to achieve a smooth consistency. While the soup is blending, add the cheese and process until smooth. Finish by adding the lemon juice, honey, salt, and pepper.
2 tablespoons lemon juice	
2 tablespoons honey	
½ teaspoon kosher salt	
½ tablespoon pepper	

Per serving: Kcalories 216 (From Fat 59); Fat 7g (Saturated 4g); Cholesterol 23mg; Sodium 324mg; Carbohydrate 28g (Dietary Fiber 3g); Protein 14g.

Choosing Chilled Soups

Chilled soups are great appetizers, light lunches, or even desserts. You can choose any taste (sweet, spicy, savory) or ethnic flavor profile (Latin, Polish, French, you name it), and there's probably a chilled soup to match. Because you serve them cold, they're great to serve all summer long.

Don't feel like you need to wait for a special occasion to serve these chilled soups. They're so easy that you can serve them any time.

Get started with chilled soups by trying the easy Chilled Cucumber Soup in this section. Spice it up as you see fit. Substitute fresh mint or cilantro for the dill to change the flavor.

Fruit soups, like the ones in this section, are among the most popular chilled soups, probably because people often eat fruit cold. So puréeing it first and then eating it isn't a stretch. Fruit soup recipes aren't always that simple, but they're not much tougher. Try cooking fruit soups with that classic blend of strawberries and rhubarb. Watermelon is the star of another recipe in this section.

Chilled Cucumber Soup

Prep time: 20 min • **Cook time:** 15 min • **Yield:** 4 servings

Ingredients	*Directions*
Nonstick cooking spray	*1* Coat a large skillet with the cooking spray and place over medium heat until hot. Sauté the cucumber and shallots, tossing or stirring frequently until soft and translucent (about 5 minutes).
1 large or 2 small cucumbers, peeled, seeded, and cut into ¼-inch slices (2 cups)	
2 shallots, minced	*2* Stir in the wine and chicken broth. Bring to a boil and simmer for 10 minutes. Add the pepper and salt. Continue to simmer for 2 minutes. Remove from heat.
¼ cup white wine	
2 cups low-sodium chicken broth	
¼ teaspoon pepper	*3* Place the contents of the skillet in an electric blender or a food processor, cover, and process until smooth.
⅛ teaspoon salt	
½ cup nonfat sour cream	*4* Pour the mixture into a bowl. Let cool slightly. With a wire whisk, stir in the sour cream and yogurt. Cover and chill. Garnish with the dill weed sprigs.
½ cup plain nonfat yogurt	
4 fresh dill weed sprigs	

Per serving: Kcalories 66 (From Fat 8); Fat 1g (Saturated 0g); Cholesterol 3mg; Sodium 186mg; Carbohydrate 10g (Dietary Fiber 1g); Protein 5g.

Tip: Make cucumber soup even more refreshing by adding naturally tart yogurt. Yogurt, plus the nonfat sour cream in this recipe, makes this soup a substantial and satisfying starter course for lunch or dinner. Or add a punch of lemon zest to create a tangy palate cleanser between courses.

Live Cucumber and Avocado Soup

Prep time: 10 min • **Yield:** 4 servings

Ingredients	*Directions*
4 cucumbers, roughly chopped	*1* In a high-speed blender combine cucumbers, avocados, jalapeño, cilantro, mint leaves, lime juice, and salt. Blend on high until all ingredients have been well puréed, about 1-2 minutes.
2 avocados, peeled and pits removed	
½ jalapeño, seeds removed	
¼ bunch cilantro	*2* Place a fine mesh strainer over a 1-2 quart container. Drain the avocado mixture through the strainer, working it through with a spatula if necessary. Taste and reseason with salt and pepper if desired.
1 sprig mint, stems removed	
Juice from ½ lime	
½ teaspoon salt	*3* Ladle a serving of the cucumber and avocado soup into a bowl. Place the julienne of radish and red bell pepper, and some sweet corn kernels on top to garnish. Enjoy!
1 small radish, julienned and chopped	
Sweet corn kernels cut from 1 ear	
½ red bell pepper, julienned and chopped	

Per serving: Kcalories 190 (Calories from Fat 118); Fat 13g (Saturated 3g); Cholesterol 0mg; Sodium 300mg; Carbohydrate 19g (Dietary Fiber 10g); Protein 5g.

Rhubarb Soup with Fresh Strawberries

Prep time: 15 min • **Cook time:** 20 min • **Yield:** 2 servings

Ingredients	Directions
1 pound rhubarb, peeled and cut into ½-inch-thick slices	*1* In a large mixing bowl, combine the rhubarb and Splenda and mix well. Set the bowl aside.
¼ cup Splenda	
1 pound strawberries, cleaned and sliced	*2* In a saucepan, combine the strawberries, water, and lemon juice. Cover and boil for 5 to 6 minutes. Using a colander, strain the strawberries to obtain just the juice. Discard the pulp.
1 cup water	
Juice of ½ lemon	
6 mint leaves, julienned	*3* Pour the strawberry juice back into the saucepan and add the rhubarb-and-Splenda mixture. Boil for 10 to 15 minutes. Remove the pan from heat and store the soup in the refrigerator until it's cold. Serve the soup chilled with the mint leaves as a garnish.

Per serving: Kcalories 117 (From Fat 10); Fat 1g (Saturated 0g); Cholesterol 0mg; Sodium 10mg; Carbohydrate 27g (Dietary Fiber 8g); Protein 3g.

Tip: Because rhubarb is seasonal, you may need to use the frozen kind, which already comes in pieces.

Watermelon Gazpacho

Prep time: 45 min • **Chill time:** 1 hr • **Yield:** 4 servings

Ingredients	Directions
1 cup thinly sliced cucumbers	**1** In a small bowl, toss the cucumbers with the salt.
¼ teaspoon kosher salt	
6 cups cubed and seeded watermelon (from about a 3-pound seedless watermelon)	**2** In a blender, add the watermelon and cranberry juice. Pulse until just blended. (Overblending causes the watermelon to froth and lose its color.) Pour through a sieve into a bowl and press on the pulp to extract all the juice. Discard the pulp.
½ cup cranberry juice	
½ cup small diced red bell pepper	**3** Add the bell pepper, onion, celery, parsley, vinegar, and lime juice to the watermelon juice. Cover and refrigerate for 1 hour to chill and allow the flavors to blend together.
½ cup small diced red onion	
½ cup small diced celery	
¼ cup finely chopped parsley	**4** Rinse the cucumbers and pat dry.
1 tablespoon sherry vinegar	
2 tablespoons lime juice	**5** Ladle the soup into chilled bowls (or martini glasses) and garnish with the cucumber slices and mint.
8 each fresh mint leaves, chiffonade (see Chapter 9 for an explanation of chiffonade)	

Per serving: Kcalories 116 (From Fat 11); Fat 1g (Saturated 0g); Cholesterol 0mg; Sodium 140mg; Carbohydrate 27g (Dietary Fiber 3g); Protein 2g.

Chapter 9

The Versatility of Salads

In This Chapter

▶ Exploring salad greens

▶ Trying out tomatoes and nuts

▶ Slipping in some fruit

▶ Including protein to complete your meal

Salads are among the most flexible items in a diabetic diet. They're chock-full of delicious and nutritious veggies with complex carbohydrates that help people with diabetes manage their glucose levels. Depending on what you add to them, dress them with, or pair them with, they can be a snack, meal, appetizer, or even a terrific last course. Stuff them in a pita pocket for a quick sandwich. Fill up a portable plastic container with them for an easy brown-bag lunch. Or toss them with a light vinaigrette for an easy meal.

In this chapter, we show you how to make the most from your salad choices. We give you excellent ideas for veggie-only salads and tips for whipping up great homemade dressings to match your nutritional needs. We show you how to add fruit to your salads for a sweet, refreshing twist. And finally, we offer recipes for entree-style, protein-packed salads, a perfect meal solution for just about any nutritional quandary.

Feasting on Great Salad Greens

Whether greens are an important part of the salad you're making or added just for garnish, using special and novel greens makes your salad stand out. Skip the pale green iceberg lettuce and buy some darker green lettuces like romaine and leaf lettuce instead (see Figure 9-1 for a sampling). The greener the leaf, the more nutrients it contains, especially magnesium, a mineral important for heart and bone health.

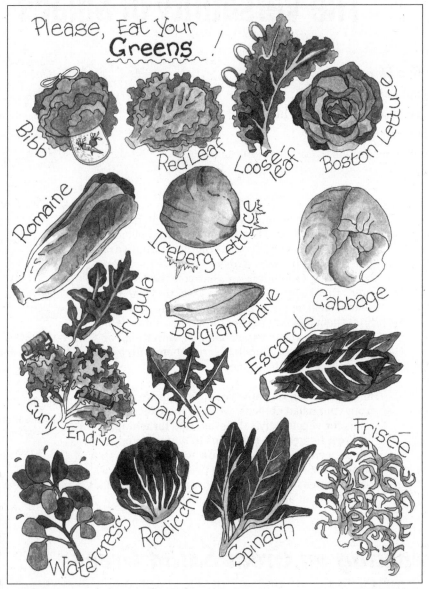

Figure 9-1:
A sampling of tasty greens to try for your next salad.

Illustration by Elizabeth Kurtzman

Picking fresh greens at the store

When you go shopping, consider picking up some of these types of greens:

- Arugula
- Boston butter lettuce
- Endive
- Escarole
- Frisée
- Mizuna
- Radicchio
- Red leaf lettuce
- Romaine
- Spinach
- Swiss chard
- Watercress

Store your salad greens in the vegetable bin of your fridge. Store romaine and radicchio with the head intact because the outer leaves keep the inner leaves moist. However, loose-leaf lettuce, like arugula and spinach, has a shorter shelf life. To store this type of lettuce, remove the leaves and wash and drain them. Gather and wrap them in a clean, damp paper towel or two and then store in a plastic bag. The leaves will stay fresh for a couple days, but not much longer.

Kale Salad

Prep time: 15 min • **Yield:** 4 servings

Ingredients	*Directions*
1 bunch kale leaves, rinsed and stems trimmed	*1* Message the kale by removing the fibrous ribs, taking bunches into both hands and rubbing together for 5 minutes. Chop the kale into thin ribbons and place in a large bowl.
2 tablespoons walnuts	
1 shallot, diced	
2 small tomatoes, cut into quarters	*2* Chop the walnuts.
4 tablespoons reduced-fat feta cheese	*3* Add the walnuts, shallot, tomatoes, feta, and dried cranberries to the kale.
1 tablespoon dried cranberries	
2 tablespoons walnut oil	*4* Toss with walnut oil and lemon juice.
2 tablespoons lemon juice	

Per serving: Kcalories 153 (From Fat 99); Fat 11g (Saturated Fat 1.5g); Cholesterol 9mg; Sodium 129mg; Carbohydrate 12g (Dietary Fiber 3g); Protein 5g.

Arugula Salad

Prep time: 10 min • **Yield:** 4 servings

Ingredients	Directions
10 to 12 ounces arugula, washed and drained	*1* Discard the arugula stems and chop the leaves into smaller pieces. Place on a serving dish.
1 or 2 garlic cloves, mashed with salt	
2 tablespoons lemon juice	*2* In a small bowl, whisk together the garlic, lemon juice, olive oil, red pepper, and salt and pepper. Pour over the arugula and toss.
3 tablespoons extra-virgin olive oil	
1 teaspoon crushed red pepper	*3* Add the tomatoes on top.
Salt and pepper to taste	
2 tomatoes, peeled and cut in bite-size pieces	

Per serving: Kcalories 111 (From Fat 99); Fat 11g (Saturated Fat 2g); Cholesterol 0mg; Sodium 14mg; Carbohydrate 4g (Dietary Fiber 2g); Protein 2g.

Watercress Salad

Prep time: 30 min • **Yield:** 4 servings

Ingredients	*Directions*

Vinaigrette dressing:

½ **onion, finely chopped**

1 teaspoon chopped fresh thyme

1 teaspoon chopped fresh oregano

¼ **cup canola oil**

¼ **cup sherry vinegar**

Salt and pepper

Salad:

2 small Granny Smith apples

8 cups watercress, rinsed, destemmed and patted dry (purchase ready-to-use watercress if time is limited)

4 ounces Gorgonzola blue cheese, crumbled

½ **cup roasted pecans (see the tip at the end of the recipe)**

1 To prepare the vinaigrette, place the onion, thyme, and oregano into a large bowl. Add the canola oil and sherry vinegar. Whisk the mixture together until everything is well combined. Add salt and pepper to taste.

2 Prepare the apples just before ready to serve to maintain their freshness and color. Leaving the skin on, slice the apples in half and core them. Julienne (slice into long strips) the cored apples.

3 Place the watercress in a large bowl and add the dressing. (You may not need all the dressing, so add carefully to taste.) Dish onto four plates and sprinkle the blue cheese and pecans over the greens. Arrange the apples on top and serve.

Per serving (with 2 tablespoons vinaigrette): Kcalories 368 (From Fat 288); Fat 32g (Saturated 8g); Cholesterol 25mg; Sodium 559mg; Carbohydrate 16g (Dietary Fiber 4g); Protein 9g.

Tip: To prepare the roasted pecans, preheat the oven to 350 degrees. Place a piece of parchment paper on a baking sheet and spread out the pecans in one even layer. Sprinkle with 1 teaspoon sugar. Bake for 10 minutes and then remove from the baking sheet. Set aside to cool.

Chili Lime Mint Vinaigrette Watermelon Salad

Prep time: 15 min • **Yield:** 8 servings

Ingredients	Directions
2 teaspoons shallots, chopped	*1* In a medium bowl, combine the shallot, Serrano, salt, lime juice, and vinegar. Let sit for 15 minutes.
½ tablespoon Serrano pepper, finely chopped	
½ teaspoon salt	*2* Whisk in the paprika, cayenne, mint, and olive oil.
2 tablespoons lime juice	*3* On 8 plates, arrange the lettuce.
2 tablespoons Champagne vinegar	*4* Top with the watermelon, cucumber, radishes, and cheese.
2 teaspoons paprika	
1 pinch cayenne	*5* Drizzle with the vinaigrette and serve.
1 tablespoon julienned mint	
½ cup light olive oil	
1 or 2 hearts of Romaine lettuce	
4 cups watermelon, cubed to 1 inch	
2 cups lemon cucumbers, peeled and cut into wedges	
1 cup radishes, sliced	
1 cup sheep's milk feta cheese, cubed	

Per serving: Kcalories 131 (From Fat 36); Fat 4g (Saturated 3g); Cholesterol 16mg; Sodium 210mg; Carbohydrate 10g (Dietary Fiber 1g); Protein 4g.

Fresh Mushroom Salad

Prep time: 20 min, plus several days for steeping the olive oil • **Yield:** 4 servings

Ingredients	Directions
1 ounce dried porcini mushrooms	*1* Prepare your own porcini olive oil by steeping the dried porcini mushrooms in the olive oil. Let stand a few days for the oil to acquire the flavor of the mushrooms. Save the oil you don't need in this recipe for future use to give any number of dishes a fabulous taste.
1 quart extra-virgin olive oil	
10 ounces fresh porcini mushrooms	
1 bunch Lolla Rossa lettuce (or substitute red leaf lettuce)	*2* Put 8 mushrooms aside and slice the remaining mushrooms very thin.
1 bunch oak leaf lettuce	
Juice of 1 lemon	*3* On 4 medium-size plates, place a few leaves of Lolla Rossa over a few oak leaf lettuce leaves. Place 1 whole mushroom on either side of the lettuce leaves to look as if the mushrooms are growing between the lettuce leaves. Place the sliced mushrooms in the remaining space on the plate.
Salt and pepper	
	4 Drizzle the porcini olive oil and lemon juice over the mushrooms and lettuce, and salt and pepper to taste.

Per serving (with 2 tablespoons porcini olive oil): Kcalories 286 (From Fat 248); Fat 28g (Saturated 4g); Cholesterol 0mg; Sodium 175mg; Carbohydrate 9g (Dietary Fiber 3g); Protein 4g.

Tip: Drizzle your extra porcini olive oil on steamed or roasted veggies, add a touch of it to risotto during the final stages of cooking, or use it to give a punch of flavor to a marinade.

Boning up on bagged salad blends

Fortunately, produce manufacturers are taking convenience foods to a healthy level for a change. Look in your produce section for prewashed, ready-to-use salad greens and blends. You can open a bag and have a delicious meal in a matter of minutes. For super easy and quick salads, pick up prewashed salad blends like these:

- ✔ **American blend:** This familiar blend usually includes iceberg lettuce, carrot shreds, radish slices, and red cabbage.

- ✔ **European blend:** It's a great mix to try if your salad experience stops at iceberg lettuce. It includes mild green leaf lettuce, romaine, iceberg, curly endive, and a bit of radicchio. It goes well with just about any dressing, toasted nuts, and any kind of cheese, including blue cheese and goat cheese.

- ✔ **Italian blend:** This blend is terrific for simple protein-based salads, light Caesar dressing, or a traditional Italian vinaigrette. It usually consists of a blend of romaine and radicchio.

- ✔ **Spring mix:** This tasty mixture is a staple at most fine restaurants. It's usually a blend of baby greens that include baby spinach, radicchio, and frisée. It may also be called mesclun, spring greens, or field greens. It makes a gorgeous garnish or bed for serving fresh fish or steak.

Different manufacturers call different mixes by different trademarked names. Many blends also include other veggies, like radishes, carrots, and even snow peas. All blends should include a description or listing of the greens (and other tasty veggies) included in their package, so find what suits your fancy and get munching!

Although these salad greens blends are great, many manufacturers also sell salad kits, which include the salad greens, dressing, cheese, and croutons. Watch the fat and unnecessary calories that these convenience kits can provide. And remember, you don't have to eat it just because it comes in the kit. Feel free to toss that full-fat Caesar dressing in the trash.

Growing your own greens

Growing fresh baby greens is incredibly simple, no matter where you live. Their shallow root systems make them ideal for indoor gardening. All you need is a shallow bowl or planter, high-quality potting soil, lettuce seeds, and a nice sunny window.

Here's how you do it:

1. **Fill a shallow container that has good drainage with high-quality potting soil.**

2. **Gently press seeds into the soil.**

   Because you'll be harvesting your baby greens when they're, well, babies, you don't need to space out the seeds. Go ahead and just sprinkle them around rather than make nice neat rows.

3. **Water your seeds.**

   Keep the seeds moist but not soggy. Light but frequent watering produces the best leafy greens.

4. **Set the container in a sunny window.**

   Most greens *germinate,* or sprout seeds, within a few weeks. Feel free to start harvesting when the greens are a few inches tall. Just trim off what you need with kitchen shears.

To keep a constant supply of greens on hand, sow a second container two weeks later. Use a mixture of different seeds to create your own spring mix. For more information on growing lettuce or other vegetables in containers, check out *Container Gardening For Dummies,* by Bill Marken and the editors of the National Gardening Association, published by Wiley.

Creating sensational homemade dressings

Until very recently, bottled salad dressings didn't offer much in the way of flavor unless they were full of fat, salt, sugar, and other no-nos for a diabetic diet. Some of the newer light dressings have improved flavor, are less detrimental to your health, and are convenient. But there's really no substitute for making dressings yourself. And believe it or not, the process is pretty simple.

To make basic diabetic-friendly vinaigrette, follow these steps:

1. **Measure equal parts oil (usually extra-virgin olive oil), acid (like balsamic vinegar or lemon juice), and stock (like low-sodium chicken stock) and whisk them together.**

2. **Blend desired herbs and seasonings into the dressing and whisk some more.**

To add a truly professional touch, combine all your ingredients (except the oil) in a food processor or blender. With the appliance running, slowly pour the oil into the other ingredients. The dressing will *emulsify,* or blend, really well.

Truffle Vinaigrette

Prep time: 5 min • **Yield:** 18–20 servings (2 tablespoons per serving)

Ingredients	*Directions*
1 to 2 ounces truffles, cleaned and finely chopped **1 small shallot, peeled and finely chopped** **3 to 4 thyme sprigs, picked and chopped** **⅓ cup balsamic vinegar** **1 cup olive oil** **Salt and pepper to taste** **Drizzle of truffle oil**	Combine all the ingredients in a bowl and whisk them together well, or combine all the ingredients in a jar with a lid and shake vigorously.

Per serving (2 tablespoons): Kcalories 105 (From Fat 99); Fat 11g (Saturated 2g); Cholesterol 0mg; Sodium 31mg; Carbohydrate 2g (Dietary Fiber 1g); Protein 0g.

Note: Often, a simple dressing is best. Steeping herbs, garlic, and dried mushrooms in oil gives you an excellent base to make your own tasty dressings. Add a little acid, like lemon juice or vinegar, and you're on your way.

Going beyond Greens with Tomatoes

For many people, salad and lettuce are synonymous. While salad greens are amazingly nutritious, it's fun to try your hand at other salads that highlight other terrific vegetables, like tomatoes and cucumbers. Flavor them up with other extras, such as toasted nuts and freshly made dressings, and you have a great alternative to a traditional salad. For another great salad without greens, check out the Olive and Lentil Salad in Chapter 10.

Getting nutty with salads

Nuts have an undeserved reputation for being fattening. Not so! In moderation, nuts are an excellent source of fiber and monounsaturated fat, the good fat. Plus, they provide you with long-lasting protein that helps to stabilize your blood sugar.

Here's a list of seeds and nuts to try in your next salad:

✔ Almonds

✔ Cashews

✔ Pecans

✔ Pine nuts

✔ Sunflower seeds

✔ Walnuts

Whenever possible, toast nuts before adding them to any dish. The toasting process really brings out the flavor of the nuts, making them much more satisfying to eat. Simply place them in a sauté pan over medium-high heat, shaking them occasionally to ensure they don't burn. They're done when they become fragrant and slightly darker in color.

Summer Tomato Salad

Prep time: 10 min • **Yield:** 4 servings

Ingredients	Directions
4 medium tomatoes, diced small	Combine all the ingredients in a large bowl and serve the salad at room temperature.
1 garlic clove, minced	
6 leaves basil, chiffonade (the sidebar "Flavoring salads with fresh herbs," later in this chapter, explains chiffonade)	
2 tablespoons olive oil	
1 tablespoon balsamic vinegar	
Salt and pepper to taste	

Per serving: Kcalories 99 (From Fat 65); Fat 7g (Saturated 1g); Cholesterol 0mg; Sodium 152mg; Carbohydrate 8g (Dietary Fiber 1g); Protein 1g.

Tip: Try a combination of tomatoes in this salad to add color and flavor. Look for Green Zebras, yellow teardrops, pear tomatoes, grape tomatoes, and everyone's first favorite tomato, the cherry. So many choices, so little time!

Salad of Imported Mozzarella di Bufala, Cherry Stem Tomatoes and Fresh Basil

Prep time: 10 min • **Yield:** 4 servings

Ingredients	Directions
24 cherry-stem tomatoes	**1** Cut the tomatoes in the middle.
12 cherry-size balls of imported Mozzarella di Bufala from Campania, Italy	**2** Repeat the process with the mozzarella balls.
1 ounce fresh basil	**3** On each of 4 plates, arrange three halved mozzarella balls and six halved cherry tomatoes.
Pepper to taste	
Kosher salt to taste	
2 tablespoons extra-virgin olive oil	**4** Season with salt and pepper. Drizzle with olive oil.
4 basil leaves, for garnish	**5** Garnish with basil leaves.

Per serving: Kcalories 288 (From Fat 225); Fat 25g (Saturated Fat 7g); Cholesterol 30mg; Sodium 60mg; Carbohydrate 0g (Dietary Fiber 0g); Protein 15g.

Flavoring salads with fresh herbs

Fresh herbs are an excellent addition to almost anything, especially salad. Their robust flavors can help you cut down the need for adding fat and salt to your foods. You can mince herbs, but some recipes, such as the one for Summer Tomato Salad in this chapter, call for herbs to be *chiffonade.* Chiffonade literally means "made of rags," and it pretty well describes what the final product looks like. Leafy lettuce or herbs are rolled together tightly and then thinly sliced width-wise to form long, stringy strips.

Here are a few descriptions of our favorite salad herbs.

✔ **Basil:** Technically a member of the mint family, this herb has a sweet peppery flavor that's the cornerstone of most pestos. Look for basil varieties like lemon basil and cinnamon basil to spice up your everyday salads.

✔ **Cilantro:** Use the tender stems and leaves of this herb to give a pungent push to any Latin- or Asian-inspired dishes. It pairs extremely well with citrus flavors.

✔ **Dill:** The feathery leaves of this pungent herb are the main ingredient in many a salad dressing and fish sauce. It's great paired with citrus.

✔ **Mint:** Sometimes thought of as only the dessert garnish, mint is used worldwide in both sweet and savory dishes. It's an incredibly aromatic herb that can lend its fragrance and flavor to salad dressings, dips, condiments, and beverages.

✔ **Parsley:** Whether you prefer flat-leaf or curly parsley, this herb is recognizable to most people. The best way to describe its flavor is fresh. Some people use it as a natural breath freshener. Chop it up and throw it into your salad along with your greens to brighten your salad's flavor.

Adding Fresh Fruit to Your Salad

Everyone knows how refreshing fruit salad can taste, made with three or four of the season's best crops. But in a diabetic diet, fruit, which is full of natural and easily absorbed sugars, needs to be enjoyed in moderation. How can you still include the juicy pleasures of fruit in a diabetic diet? By creating meals with small amounts of fruit and combining it with other foods, as in the following Fig, Mozzarella, and Mizuna Salad. Figs, mozzarella, and olive oil combine to balance the fat, protein, and carbohydrates.

Fig, Mozzarella, and Mizuna Salad with Thai Basil

Prep time: 15 min • **Yield:** 4 servings

Ingredients	Directions
8 green figs	*1* Wash the figs and remove the little stems with a paring knife. Remove the mozzarella balls from their liquid. Wash the greens; drain thoroughly. Remove basil (or mint if using) leaves from the stems. Wash the herbs; pat the leaves dry.
12 small balls of fresh mozzarella	
1 bunch or 12 ounces mizuna or arugula	
1 bunch or 4 ounces Thai basil or purple mint	*2* Place the greens and herbs in a medium bowl and toss with the olive oil.
⅓ cup fruity extra-virgin olive oil	*3* Pile the greens mixture in the middle of four dinner plates. Using your thumbs, gently pull figs in half and lay them open-side up around the greens mixture on the plates. Arrange 3 balls of cheese around the greens pile on each plate well.
1 teaspoon coarse salt	
Freshly ground black pepper, to taste	
	4 Sprinkle each plate with a little extra olive oil, a few drops of lemon juice, and a sprinkle of coarse salt. Grind fresh pepper to taste over each salad.

Per serving: Kcalories 428 (Calories from Fat 286); Fat 32g (Saturated 11g); Cholesterol 47mg; Sodium 824mg; Carbohydrate 25g (Dietary Fiber 6g); Protein 15g.

Note: Mizuna is a Japanese mustard green. Its leaves are shaped much like dandelion leaves, but are more subtle and delicate, with a jagged edge, and a mild earthy flavor. It's a great lettuce to grow yourself, so if you can't find it in a gourmet grocery store near you, consider growing your own with the instructions later in this chapter.

Enjoying Entree Salads

For many of us, salads have become the main attraction. These days you can even get a very decent entree salad at your local fast food restaurant. Eating salad has never been easier. To continue that push toward easy healthful eating, we offer you the tasty entree salads in this section.

Surveying simple seafood salads

Most seafood is naturally delicious, so it really doesn't take much effort to turn it into something special. A little bit of seasoning, a light dressing, and some tasty greens, and you have yourself a meal. Marinate sea scallops in a little olive oil and lemon juice and broil them. Or steam your favorite white fish with herbs and seasonings and then serve it on a bed of greens. Just about any seafood item can take the main stage in your mostly salad meal. For more terrific seafood recipes, make sure to stop by Chapter 12.

Shrimp Salad

Prep time: 15 min • **Yield:** 4 servings

Ingredients	*Directions*
1 pound medium shrimp, cooked	*1* In a bowl, combine the shrimp, red and yellow bell peppers, half of the cilantro, and chives.
¼ cup chopped red bell pepper	
¼ cup chopped yellow bell pepper	*2* In another bowl, whisk together the mayonnaise, mustard, lemon juice, and white pepper. Spoon over the shrimp mixture and toss together.
1 tablespoon chopped fresh cilantro	
¼ cup chopped fresh chives	*3* Arrange the salad greens on 4 large plates. Top the greens with equal portions of the shrimp mixture.
¼ cup lowfat mayonnaise	
1 teaspoon Dijon mustard	*4* Sprinkle with the remaining cilantro.
1 teaspoon lemon juice	
¼ teaspoon white pepper	
4 cups fresh mixed salad greens	

Per serving: Kcalories 154 (From Fat 23); Fat 3g (Saturated 0g); Cholesterol 221mg; Sodium 440mg; Carbohydrate 7g (Dietary Fiber 2g); Protein 25g.

Punching up your salad with protein

Pairing salads and protein is a natural fit for a diabetic diet. Most of the meal is actually made up of the healthy veggies, accented by a small but satisfying portion of protein, the ideal ratio in a diabetic diet.

Canned legumes, like chickpeas (also known as garbanzo beans) and kidney beans, are an excellent and inexpensive way to make sure you're getting enough protein. Plus these protein powerhouses are cholesterol free, making them an all-around excellent choice.

Chickpea Salad

Prep time: 10 min • **Yield:** 2 servings

Ingredients	*Directions*
1½ cups canned chickpeas, drained and rinsed	*1* In a bowl, coarsely mash the chickpeas. Add the celery, red pepper, onion, salt, pepper, and mayonnaise and toss well.
¼ cup celery, chopped	
¼ cup red bell pepper, chopped	*2* Serve over pita bread or mixed greens.
¼ cup red onion, chopped	
⅛ teaspoon salt	
⅛ teaspoon white pepper	
2 tablespoons lowfat mayonnaise	
Pita bread or mixed greens	

Per serving (without pita or greens): Kcalories 206 (From Fat 30); Fat 3g (Saturated 0g); Cholesterol 0mg; Sodium 641mg; Carbohydrate 35g (Dietary Fiber 9g); Protein 10g.

Note: This great, all-purpose salad can be stuffed in a pita pocket with mixed greens for a quick well-rounded meal. Vary it by adding different vegetables, like tomatoes, or different spices, like cumin or curry powder. Make it your own.

Crunchy Chicken Stir-Fry Salad

Prep time: 15 min • **Cook time:** 25 min • **Yield:** 2 servings

Ingredients	Directions
1 tablespoon sesame oil	*1* Heat a large skillet over medium-high heat. Add the oil. Add the chicken strips, carrots, and garlic powder. Sauté until the chicken is lightly browned (about 7 minutes). Add the onion powder, white pepper, sesame seeds, broccoli, and celery. Cook and continue stirring until the vegetables are soft.
12 ounces boneless, skinless chicken breasts, sliced into strips	
½ cup baby carrots	
¼ teaspoon garlic powder	
⅛ teaspoon onion powder	*2* Lower the heat and add the snap peas, teriyaki sauce, soy sauce, and chicken broth. Continue stirring. Simmer until the liquid has reduced slightly.
⅛ teaspoon white pepper	
¼ teaspoon sesame seeds	
½ cup broccoli florets	*3* Divide the bok choy between two plates. Spoon the chicken mixture over the bok choy. Sprinkle the almonds on top.
¼ cup celery, small sliced diagonally	
½ cup snap peas	
1 tablespoon low-sodium teriyaki sauce	
1 teaspoon low-sodium soy sauce	
½ cup low-sodium chicken broth	
1 cup blanched and roughly chopped Chinese bok choy (see Chapter 11 for info about blanching)	
2 tablespoons slivered almonds	

Per serving: Kcalories 352 (From Fat 136); Fat 15g (Saturated 3g); Cholesterol 95mg; Sodium 403mg; Carbohydrate 12g (Dietary Fiber 5g); Protein 40g.

Egg Salad with Hummus

Prep time: 20 min • **Yield:** 6 servings

Ingredients	Directions
6 hard-boiled eggs	**1** Peel and slice the eggs in half lengthwise. Remove the yolks.
¼ cup classic hummus	
1 teaspoon Dijon mustard	**2** In a medium bowl, combine the egg yolks with all the other ingredients.
1 teaspoon yellow mustard	
½ tablespoon yellow curry powder	
½ lemon juiced	
1 cup fresh, washed kale, chopped	
Salt and pepper to taste	

Per serving: Kcalories 177 (From Fat 90); Fat 10g (Saturated Fat 2g); Cholesterol 186mg; Sodium 177mg; Carbohydrate 5g (Dietary Fiber 1g); Protein 8g.

Using leftovers to your advantage

"Leftovers" doesn't have to be a dirty word. In fact, think of them as a life simplification strategy. When you're marinating and grilling chicken for dinner, double your recipe and reserve the extra for quick salads later in the week. Stop by the grocery on your way home and get a fresh bag of greens, and your healthful dinner is in the bag.

Here's a list of great leftovers that can make an excellent next-day salad:

- ✔ Broiled sirloin steak
- ✔ Grilled chicken breast
- ✔ Cocktail shrimp
- ✔ Roasted turkey breast
- ✔ Pan-seared beef tenderloin
- ✔ Roasted pork tenderloin

Oriental Beef and Noodle Salad

Prep time: 15 min • **Cook time:** 15 min • **Yield:** 4 servings

Ingredients	*Directions*
8 ounces thin spaghetti	*1* Bring a large pot of water to boil. Salt the boiling water and cook the spaghetti according to package directions, typically 5 to 6 minutes. Drain, rinse under cold running water, and drain again. Transfer to a large bowl and toss with the sesame oil and set aside.
4 teaspoons sesame oil	
Nonstick cooking spray	
1 pound boneless top sirloin steak, trimmed of fat, cut 1-inch thick, and cut into slices about ¼-inch thick	*2* Coat a large cast-iron or nonstick skillet with the cooking spray and place over medium-high heat until hot. Add the steak slices and cook until medium rare, about 1 minute per side. Add the steak to the bowl with the pasta.
2 teaspoons low-sodium soy sauce	
2 teaspoons red wine vinegar	*3* In a small bowl, whisk together the soy sauce, vinegar, mustard, ginger, garlic, and white pepper. Add the green onions and red bell pepper and toss well. Add to the bowl with the spaghetti and steak and toss well.
1 teaspoon Dijon mustard	
¼ teaspoon ground ginger	
1 clove garlic, minced	
⅛ teaspoon white pepper	
2 tablespoons thinly sliced green onion	*4* Divide among four serving plates, sprinkle with the cilantro, and serve.
2 tablespoons finely chopped red bell pepper	
2 teaspoons chopped fresh cilantro	

Per serving: Kcalories 435 (From Fat 122); Fat 14g (Saturated 4g); Cholesterol 71mg; Sodium 186mg; Carbohydrate 44g (Dietary Fiber 2g); Protein 34g.

Chapter 10

Stocking Up on Grains and Legumes

Diabetics must watch their intake of carbohydrates because they directly impact blood sugar levels. One big source of carbohydrates is grains. Grains form a part of MyPlate, the guide to healthy eating from the United States Department of Agriculture (USDA). (See Chapter 2 for more about MyPlate.) Talk to your doctor and dietitian about the best choice for your health situation.

In this chapter, we show you how to include rice and other grains in recipes and dishes to brighten up any meal. We provide recipes and information on using pasta as part of your daily regimen. And finally, we give you the inside scoop on using legumes in so many ways that you're bound to find something new and tasty.

Relishing Rice and Other Grains

Grains are truly the food that changed the world. Cultivated by early farmers, they helped our ancestors become settled, non-nomadic peoples, building stable civilizations the world over. We owe a lot to these little packets of nutrition, like rice and quinoa.

Eating rice the right way

Rice is a worldwide staple, but it often gets a bad reputation because so many people eat the bland, processed white rice slathered with fat-heavy sauces. Instead, try less processed, flavored rice that can stand on its own or can be enhanced by a few simple seasonings or cooking techniques. And always remember to eat in moderation.

Here are a few rice varieties that may be new to you with ideas on how to use them:

✔ **Arborio:** It's an Italian short- to medium-grained rice used in making risotto. The rice gives off starches as it cooks to add to the creaminess of this popular Italian dish. Try it for yourself in the recipe for Risotto alle Erbe Made with Extra-Virgin Olive Oil in this section.

✔ **Basmati:** Its name means "queen of fragrance" for its distinct nutty aroma during cooking. Its fragrance is enhanced as it's aged after harvesting. True basmati rice is grown in the foothills of the Himalayas, but a few new basmati-like varieties are grown in the United States under the names Texmati and Kasmati.

✔ **Brown:** This rice has the whole rice grain intact, with only the inedible outer husk removed. Because it has the bran coating intact, it's higher in fiber but has a shorter shelf life (around six months). Use it in any recipe that calls for white rice, but give it a bit more time to cook (about 45 minutes). To get started with it, try the Middle Eastern Brown Rice Pilaf in this section.

✔ **Jasmine:** Aromatic long-grain rice from Thailand, this rice is highly prized but less expensive than basmati. Try it out in the Black Bean Pie recipe later in this chapter.

✔ **Long-grain:** A broad category of rice, long-grain rice has long, evenly shaped pieces that tend to be drier and less starchy than short-grained varieties. Long-grain rice separates easily after cooking. Basmati, jasmine, and wild rice are all long-grain rices.

✔ **Medium-grain:** As the name implies, medium-grain rice is longer than short-grain rice and shorter than long-grain rice.

✔ **Short-grain:** This rice has short, almost round grains and a higher starch content than long-grain rice, giving it a sticky, clumpy consistency after cooking.

✔ **Wild rice:** This "rice" is actually the grain of a wild marsh grass. It has a chewy texture and nutty flavor. It's often combined with other rice.

Middle Eastern Brown Rice Pilaf

Prep time: 10 min • **Cook time:** 1 hr • **Yield:** 6 servings

Ingredients	Directions
2 tablespoons olive oil	*1* Heat the olive oil in a deep skillet with a tight-fitting lid over medium heat. Sauté the onions, stirring frequently until they soften. Add the garlic and carrots and continue stirring for 5 minutes. Add the mushrooms and rice and cook until the mushrooms soften, about 7 to 8 minutes.
1½ cups chopped onion	
1 clove garlic, minced	
2 carrots, sliced	
2 cups fresh sliced mushrooms	
¾ cup uncooked brown rice	*2* Add the chicken broth. Bring to a boil. Cover and reduce the heat. Continue cooking until all the liquid is absorbed, approximately 45 to 50 minutes. Fluff with a fork. Toss with the green onions. Season with salt and pepper to taste.
2 cups chicken broth	
¼ cup chopped fresh green onions	
Salt and pepper	

Per serving: Kcalories 174 (From Fat 60); Fat 7g (Saturated 1g); Cholesterol 2mg; Sodium 547mg; Carbohydrate 25g (Dietary Fiber 3g); Protein 4g.

Risotto alle Erbe Made with Extra-Virgin Olive Oil

Prep time: 45 min • **Cook time:** 20 min • **Yield:** 6 servings (1 cup each)

Ingredients	Directions
1 bunch fresh sage	*1* From the fresh sage, rosemary, parsley, and basil, chop enough in equal parts (roughly 3 tablespoons) of each type of herb to make ¾ cup. Set aside.
1 bunch fresh rosemary	
1 bunch fresh parsley	
1 bunch fresh basil	*2* Using butcher's twine, tie together one stem each of sage, rosemary, parsley, and basil (once tied together, the herbs resemble a bouquet of flowers). Place the bouquet in a saucepan with the 1½ quarts of water. Bring to a boil. Remove from heat. Allow the bouquet to steep for 30 minutes. Strain and keep warm. This will serve as your herb stock. Bring stock back to a low simmer before adding to risotto in Step 4.
1½ quarts water	
5 tablespoons extra-virgin olive oil, divided	
½ medium onion, finely chopped	
1 teaspoon salt	
Pinch of pepper	*3* In a 3-quart saucepan, heat 3 tablespoons of oil over medium heat. Add the chopped onions, salt, and pepper. Cook for 1 minute. Add the rice, wine, and chopped herbs. Immediately stir and continue to stir every 15 seconds until the risotto absorbs the wine. Keep the heat medium to high. When the wine has evaporated, begin to add simmering stock ½ cup at time, stirring continuously. Add a bit of salt and pepper depending on your taste. Once ½ cup of the stock is absorbed and the rice looks dry, add another ½ cup. Repeat until you've added roughly 3 to 4 cups of the herb stock, and the rice is soft but *al dente,* or firm to the bite. If the rice tastes hard and starchy, continue adding stock. This step takes about 25 to 30 minutes total. ***Note:*** You must continue to stir the risotto during this stage of cooking.
1 cup Italian rice, Carnaroti or arborio	
1 cup dry white wine	
½ cup grated Parmigiano cheese	
Salt and pepper to taste	
	4 When the risotto is cooked, its consistency should resemble thick oatmeal. Remove the pot from the heat. Add the grated Parmigiano cheese and the remaining 2 tablespoons of oil. Stir well. Allow to rest 2 minutes. Stir once more before serving. Season with salt and pepper.

Per serving: *Kcalories 278 (From Fat 128); Fat 14g (Saturated 3g); Cholesterol 5mg; Sodium 516mg; Carbohydrate 31g (Dietary Fiber 1g); Protein 7g.*

Butternut Squash Risotto

Prep time: 45 min • **Cook time:** 45 min • **Yield:** 6 servings

Ingredients	*Directions*
1 butternut squash peeled, seeded, and cut into ¾-inch cubes	*1* Preheat the oven to 400 degrees.
2½ tablespoons olive oil	*2* On a sheet pan, place the squash and toss with 1 tablespoon of the olive oil, the salt, and the pepper. Roast for 25 to 30 minutes.
1 teaspoon salt	
½ teaspoon pepper	*3* In a saucepan, heat the chicken stock and simmer.
6 cups chicken stock (Knorr gel stock if you don't have homemade)	*4* In a saucepan, sauté the shallots in the remaining 1½ tablespoons of olive oil for 10 minutes, until the white part is translucent but not browned.
½ cup chopped shallots	
1½ cups Arborio rice	*5* Add the rice and stir to coat with the olive oil.
½ cup dry white wine	*6* Add the wine to the shallots and cook for two minutes.
½ cup freshly grated Parmesan cheese	
	7 Add 1 cup of the warm stock to the rice. Stir and simmer until it's absorbed. Repeat until all the stock is used.
	8 Continue cooking for about 30 minutes, until the rice is cooked.
	9 Turn off the heat and add the roasted squash cubes and Parmesan cheese. Mix well.

Per serving: Kcalories 171 (From Fat 32); Fat 3.5g (Saturated 1g); Cholesterol 5mg; Sodium 517mg; Carbohydrate 29g (Dietary Fiber 1.5g); Protein 4.5g.

Vary It! This recipe calls for butternut squash, but you can substitute pumpkin, acorn, or another firm-fleshed squash. If you want an even more special taste, try adding 2 teaspoons chopped fresh rosemary.

Kicking it up with quinoa

Quinoa (pronounced keen-wah) is considered by some to be the most nutritious of all the whole grains (see Figure 10-1). This ancient superfood is becoming more popular, showing up on the menus of gourmet restaurants nationwide. Quinoa is high in protein and fiber, provides 25 percent of your daily iron needs, and is a tremendous source of magnesium, potassium, and phosphorus. It is more nutritious than white rice and in most dishes can be substituted for the more popular grain.

Most mainstream grocery stores carry it these days, but if you have trouble tracking it down, try your local health food store. Whenever possible, opt for the grain itself, rather than a processed boxed quinoa pilaf. As with other grains, the less processed the better.

Always rinse quinoa thoroughly before cooking it. Don't be tempted to skip this step. Even if your quinoa is processed, which removes much of the *saponin*, or protective outer covering, the dust still remains. It can add a nasty bitter flavor to your finished dish. Don't risk it. Place the quinoa in a fine mesh strainer. Run cold water through the grains until the water runs clear. Drain the water off, stir the grains around a bit, and then re-rinse to ensure you've removed all the bitter outer coating.

Figure 10-1:
Quinoa is a terrific source of protein, fiber, vitamins, and minerals.

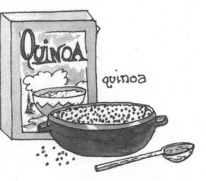

Illustration by Elizabeth Kurtzman

Moroccan Quinoa

Prep time: 20 min • **Cook time:** 40 min • **Yield:** 4 servings

Ingredients	Directions
1 cup quinoa, drained and rinsed thoroughly	*1* Place the rinsed quinoa, water, and chicken broth in a 1½-quart saucepan and bring to a boil. Reduce to a simmer, cover, and cook until all the water is absorbed (about 15 minutes). Fluff with a fork. Set aside.
1 cup water	
1 cup low-sodium chicken broth	
2 teaspoons olive oil	*2* While the quinoa is cooking, heat the oil in a nonstick skillet. Sauté the onions until they begin to caramelize. Add the cumin, turmeric, cinnamon, and ginger, cooking until fragrant. Stir in the almonds and raisins until heated.
1 cup diced red onion	
½ teaspoon cumin	
¼ teaspoon turmeric	
½ teaspoon cinnamon	*3* Add the hot quinoa to the skillet. Toss to combine. Heat until the mixture is heated through. Adjust salt if needed. Serve garnished with fresh mint, if desired.
¼ teaspoon ground ginger	
¼ cup slivered almonds, toasted	
¼ cup raisins	
Salt to taste	
Fresh mint (optional)	

Per serving: Kcalories 274 (From Fat 79); Fat 9g (Saturated 1g); Cholesterol 1mg; Sodium 186mg; Carbohydrate 43g (Dietary Fiber 5g); Protein 9g.

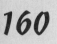

Quinoa and Black Bean Salad over Chilled Avocado Soup

Prep time: 30 min • **Cook time:** 20 min • **Cool time:** 2 hr • **Yield:** 4 servings

Ingredients	Directions
Avocado Soup:	**1** Place the ingredients for the avocado soup (except salt) into a blender. Blend until smooth. Season to taste with salt. Refrigerate until needed, at least 2 hours.
2 ripe avocados, peeled and seeded	
½ yellow onion, diced	
1 clove garlic, peeled	
½ serrano or jalapeño pepper, or more to taste	
3 tablespoons cilantro leaves	
½ teaspoon dried oregano	**2** Place the rinsed quinoa and water in a 1½-quart saucepan and bring to a boil. Reduce to a simmer, cover, and cook until all the water is absorbed (about 15 minutes). Fluff with a fork. Set aside. Allow to cool to room temperature, about an hour.
2 cups water	
Juice of 2 limes	
Salt to taste	
Quinoa Black Bean Salad:	
1 cup quinoa, rinsed and drained thoroughly	**3** Mix remaining ingredients together in a mixing bowl. Adjust salt and pepper to taste.
2 cups water	
2 15-ounce cans black beans, drained and rinsed	
½ red onion, small diced	**4** To serve, pack 1 cup of the quinoa salad into a ring mold in the center of a pasta bowl. If you don't have a ring mold handy, just mound the salad in the center of the bowl. Gently pour 3 ounces of the avocado soup around the salad.
1 cup cherry tomatoes, sliced in half	
2 tablespoons minced cilantro	
2 tablespoons minced fresh parsley	
½ teaspoon dried oregano (or 1 teaspoon fresh oregano minced)	
½ teaspoon smoked paprika	
Juice of 1 lime	
Salt and black pepper to taste	

Per serving: Kcalories 416 (Calories from Fat 160); Fat 18g (Saturated 3g); Cholesterol 0mg; Sodium 314mg; Carbohydrate 56g (Dietary Fiber 16g); Protein 15g.

Tip: No need to mince the garlic or peppers for the avocado soup. Just plop them into the blender as-is.

Cyprus Bulgur Wheat Salad

Prep time: 45 min • **Yield:** 4 servings

Ingredients	Directions
½ cup cracked bulgur wheat cooked	**1** In a medium bowl, place the bulgur.
3 bunches cilantro, shredded 5 tomatoes, deseeded and finely diced	**2** In a small bowl, mix the tomatoes, cilantro, scallions, red onion, lemon zest, lemon juice, and olive oil. Add to the bowl with the bulgur.
1 bunch scallions, finely chopped	**3** Season with salt and eat right away.
½ red onion, finely chopped	
½ lemon, zested	
2 lemons, juiced	
¼ cup olive oil	
Salt to taste	

Per serving: Kcalories 253 (From Fat 126); Fat 14g (Saturated Fat 2g); Cholesterol 0mg; Sodium 13mg; Carbohydrate 31g (Dietary Fiber 5g); Protein 5g.

Roasted Root Vegetables and Quinoa

Prep time: 30 min • **Cook time:** 45 min • **Yield:** 4 servings

Ingredients	Directions
2 medium carrots, peeled and cut into 2-inch pieces	**1** Preheat oven to 325 degrees.
2 parsnips, peeled and cut into small chunks	**2** In a large mixing bowl, place the carrots, parsnips, beets, yam, and garlic. Add remaining ingredients (except water and quinoa) to the bowl. Toss well to combine. Transfer vegetable mixture to a shallow baking sheet and bake for 45 minutes, or until tender. Add salt and pepper to taste.
2 beets, peeled and cut into small chunks	
1 yam, peeled and cut into small chunks	
1 garlic clove, sliced	**3** Meanwhile, place the rinsed quinoa and water in a 1½-quart saucepan and bring to a boil. Reduce to a simmer, cover, and cook until all the water is absorbed (about 15 minutes). Fluff with a fork.
1 tablespoon extra-virgin olive oil	
1 tablespoon soy sauce or tamari	
Pinch of dried basil	**4** To serve, mound 1 cup of quinoa in the center of plate. Ring with ¼ of the vegetables.
Pinch of dried oregano	
Pinch of dried thyme	
Pinch of freshly ground black pepper	
Salt and pepper to taste	
3 cups water	
1½ cups quinoa, rinsed and drained	

Per serving: Kcalories 418 (Calories from Fat 67); Fat 7g (Saturated 1g); Cholesterol 0mg; Sodium 308mg; Carbohydrate 79g (Dietary Fiber 11g); Protein 12g.

Tip: If you need a protein boost, consider adding a portion of grilled chicken or shrimp to this already complete meal.

Preparing Perfect Pasta

Pasta comes in many shapes and sizes. Here are some guidelines to help you decide what works for your recipe:

- ✔ For lighter, brothy sauces and pestos, choose delicate, long pasta, like vermicelli, spaghetti, linguine, or angel hair.

- ✔ For meatier, chunkier sauces or pasta salads, choose shorter shapes with ridges or holes, like cavatelli, penne, farfalle, and wagon wheels. The smaller pieces make it easier to grab pasta and sauce with every bite. And the ridges and holes in the pasta grab bits and chunks of your sauce.

- ✔ For heavier and creamier sauces, choose flat, ribbonlike pasta, such as fettuccine.

Most pasta is made from semolina flour, not refined white flour. It's a complex carbohydrate, rather than a simple carbohydrate, meaning that it gives your body more lasting energy and a more gradual release of sugar. A ½ cup serving of cooked pasta contains 99 calories, less than half a gram of fat, and less than 5 milligrams of sodium, and it costs you only 1 starch exchange.

Here are a few other benefits of choosing pasta.

- ✔ It has a relatively low glycemic index of 41. For more about the glycemic index and how it can help you manage your blood glucose levels, check out Chapter 2.

- ✔ It's a quick food to prepare. You can get this filling side dish ready in about 10 minutes.

- ✔ It goes with just about anything. Pasta is so versatile. You can toss it with chicken broth and fresh herbs, or fresh veggies and a little bit of olive oil. If you can cook it, you can serve it with pasta.

  - Create Chinese flavored dishes with a splash of sesame oil, crunchy water chestnuts, bok choy, and cilantro. Add thinly sliced beef for a full meal.

  - Mix up a Mediterranean delight by adding tomatoes, garlic, and fresh basil. Throw in some pine nuts and seafood for a lowfat, tasty weeknight supper.

  - Invent your own Latin lunch, by including grilled onions, chicken breast, chilies, and chayote squash.

  - Introduce flavors from the Caribbean by tossing pasta with shrimp, flaked coconut, jerk seasonings, and vegetable stock.

  - Work in some Vietnamese inspired cuisine, by adding it to vegetable broth, chopped chilies, cilantro, and lean pork.

✔ It's very filling. A ½ cup serving may not seem like much, but a little can go a long way, especially if you bulk up the fiber content of your dish with fresh veggies. Or opt for 2 starch servings, and have a full cup of pasta and enjoy it as a main course.

Although most of the pasta you'll find in your local grocery is made from semolina flour, you can find pasta made from a variety of different flours, including these:

✔ **Brown rice:** This pasta is a great alternative for people allergic to wheat. Check the label, but most brown rice pasta is both wheat and gluten free. They may also be dairy-free and organic. Try this delicious pasta in the following recipe.

✔ **Soy:** Pasta made with soy flour tends to be higher in protein and lower in carbohydrate than semolina pasta, but always read the label to make sure you're making the right choice for your needs.

✔ **Whole wheat:** If you're looking for a higher fiber pasta, whole-wheat pasta may be what you're looking for. It's characterized by a more robust flavor than its semolina counterpart.

Seafood Farfalle Salad

Prep time: 25 min • **Cook time:** 20–25 min • **Yield:** 4 servings

Ingredients	Directions
8 ounces farfalle pasta	**1** Bring a large pot of water to a boil. Salt the boiling water and cook the farfalle according to package directions. Drain, rinse under cold running water, and drain again. Set aside.
Nonstick cooking spray	
½ pound bay scallops	
½ pound cooked baby shrimp	**2** Meanwhile, coat a medium nonstick skillet with cooking spray or 2 teaspoons of canola oil and place over medium heat until hot. Add the scallops and shrimp, a few at a time, and sauté, turning them as they brown, allowing 1½ to 2 minutes per side; remove them to a bowl as they finish.
½ teaspoons white wine vinegar	
1 tablespoon extra-virgin olive oil	
1 teaspoon freshly squeezed lemon juice	**3** In a large bowl, whisk together the vinegar, olive oil, lemon juice, thyme, garlic, parsley, and pepper. Add the tomatoes, cucumber, and green bell pepper and mix thoroughly. Combine the pasta, scallops (and their released juices), and shrimp. Toss the pasta mixture with the dressing mixture.
1 teaspoon dried thyme leaves	
1 clove garlic, minced	
2 teaspoons chopped fresh parsley	
⅛ teaspoon black pepper	
½ cup plum tomatoes, peeled, seeded, and diced	
1 small cucumber, peeled, seeded, and diced	
2 tablespoons seeded and finely chopped green bell pepper	

Per serving: Kcalories 350 (From Fat 61); Fat 7g (Saturated 1g); Cholesterol 82mg; Sodium 167mg; Carbohydrate 47g (Dietary Fiber 3g); Protein 26g.

Letting Legumes into Your Diet

Legumes (pronounced LAY-gooms) are the protein-packed staple of a vegetarian diet, but you don't have to swear off meat to enjoy them. The family of grains includes thousands of plant species, including beans, soybeans, lentils, peas, and the beloved peanut.

It's tough to find a more perfect all-round food than legumes. They're rich in protein, low in fat (what fat they do have is the good fat), high in dietary fiber, and rich in complex carbohydrates and vitamins. Besides being healthy, they're inexpensive, very versatile, and easy to use. They store well when dried, and have a shelf life of a full year.

Because legumes are also high in carbohydrate, a person with diabetes still needs to be mindful of portion sizes here. The benefits that the fiber and protein provide, however, make them a more optimal choice than the usual carbs like bread, pasta, or rice.

Red-Wine-Braised Lentils

Prep time: 10 min • **Cook time:** 1 hr 20 min • **Yield:** 6 servings

Ingredients	Directions
1 tablespoon butter	**1** In a medium saucepan, heat the butter and olive oil. Sauté the onions, celery, and carrots, until they begin to *sweat*, or give off a bit of liquid. Season the vegetables with salt and pepper to taste and cover the pot. Cook until the vegetables are soft, approximately 10 minutes.
2 tablespoons olive oil	
1 cup diced onions	
½ cup chopped celery	
½ cup diced carrots	
Salt and pepper	**2** Add the thyme, prosciutto, and dried porcini mushrooms. Add the wine and reduce by one-third. Add the lentils, bay leaf, and chicken broth and simmer for about 1 hour, until the lentils are soft.
½ teaspoon thyme leaves	
2 ounces diced prosciutto	
¼ cup dried porcini mushrooms, reconstituted and sliced (see the tip at the end of the recipe)	**3** Remove the bay leaf. Adjust the salt and pepper if needed. This dish may be refrigerated for up to 3 days, until ready to use.
1½ cups red wine	
2 cups dried brown lentils	
1 bay leaf	
5 cups low-sodium chicken broth	

Per serving: Kcalories 348 (From Fat 88); Fat 10g (Saturated 3g); Cholesterol 17mg; Sodium 387mg; Carbohydrate 44g (Dietary Fiber 16g); Protein 23g.

Tip: To reconstitute the dried porcini mushrooms, place them in ¼ cup hot water for 30 minutes, chop them, and strain the liquid. If you want, you can use the liquid as part of the cooking liquid. Just substitute the mushroom broth for ¼ cup of the chicken broth in Step 2.

Tip: Lentils are quick cooking legumes, so you don't need to soak them before cooking like you do with dried beans. If you're extra conscientious, feel free to pick over the lentils, as you would with dried beans. Rinse them well to remove any dirt or other debris. Then sort through them a handful at a time, looking for dirt clods, stones, and other foreign particles. Try them in soups, saucy Indian curries, or this terrific "salad."

Olive and Lentil Salad

Prep time: 30 min • **Cook time:** 40 min • **Yield:** 6 servings

Ingredients	Directions

Ingredients

Salad:

1 cup dry lentils

2 bay leaves

1 sprig fresh thyme

1 carrot, finely chopped

1 stalk celery, finely chopped

2 tablespoons minced shallots

1 tablespoon minced garlic

2 Roma tomatoes, seeded and sliced thinly

½ yellow bell pepper, diced

1 jar (8 ounces) green olives, roughly chopped (reserve juice for the dressing)

2 tablespoons roughly chopped fresh oregano

Salt and pepper

4 ounces goat cheese, crumbled

Dressing:

¼ cup red wine vinegar

2 tablespoons green olive juice

1 tablespoon minced shallot

3 teaspoons Dijon mustard

1 teaspoon salt

1 teaspoon pepper

¼ cup olive oil

Directions

1 In a 2-quart saucepan, combine the lentils, bay leaves, thyme, carrots, celery, shallots, and garlic. Cover with 2 inches of water. Bring to a low boil and cook until the lentils are just tender, about 40 minutes. Drain and set aside to cool.

2 After the lentils have cooled, add the tomatoes, peppers, olives, and oregano. Mix thoroughly. Salt and pepper to taste. Gently stir in the goat cheese.

3 In a blender, combine the vinegar, olive juice, shallot, mustard, salt, and pepper. Remove the knob from the lid of the blender. With the blender running, slowly pour in the olive oil to emulsify the dressing. Adjust seasonings as necessary. Pour over the salad and toss gently to coat.

Per serving: Kcalories 343 (From Fat 192); Fat 21g (Saturated 5g); Cholesterol 15mg; Sodium 1,326mg; Carbohydrate 28g (Dietary Fiber 8g); Protein 14g.

White Beans and Spinach

Prep time: 10 min • **Cook time:** 20 min • **Yield:** 4 servings

Ingredients	Directions
1 tablespoon olive oil ½ cup diced onions 3 cloves garlic, peeled and sliced thinly 1 cup sliced cremini mushrooms ¼ cup white wine 1 tablespoon Dijon mustard	*1* Heat the olive oil in a skillet over medium-high heat. Add the onions and sauté until translucent. Add the garlic and mushrooms. Cook until just fragrant. Add the white wine and mustard. Scrape up any browned bits that may be stuck to the skillet.
Half a 10-ounce bag of triple-washed spinach 1 can (15 ounces) white beans (like navy, cannellini, or great Northern), rinsed and drained 2 tablespoons fresh minced oregano Salt and pepper	*2* Add the spinach and cover. Steam the spinach for 3 to 4 minutes, or until wilted but still bright green. Add the white beans. Continue to cook until heated through. Add the oregano and salt and pepper to taste. Adjust seasonings as necessary.

Per serving: Kcalories 122 (From Fat 37); Fat 4g (Saturated 1g); Cholesterol 0mg; Sodium 385mg; Carbohydrate 18g (Dietary Fiber 5g); Protein 5g.

Black Bean Pie

Prep time: 45 min • **Cook time:** 20 min • **Yield:** 6 servings

Ingredients	Directions
1 can (14 ounces) black beans ½ cup jasmine rice, uncooked	*1* Preheat the oven to 350 degrees. Drain the black beans and reserve the juice. Set aside.
1 9-inch frozen pie shell Nonstick cooking spray ½ cup diced onion	*2* Cook the jasmine rice according to package directions. Set aside. While the rice is cooking, bake the pie shell until slightly browned, approximately 5 to 7 minutes. Set aside.
¼ cup diced red bell pepper ¼ cup diced green bell pepper 1 tablespoon chopped fresh cilantro	*3* Heat a medium skillet over medium-high heat. Once it's heated, spray with the cooking spray. Add the onions and red and green bell peppers. Sauté until the vegetables are crisp-tender, approximately 5 to 7 minutes. Set aside.
1 teaspoon garlic powder 1 teaspoon cumin, ground 1 teaspoon chili powder ½ teaspoon cayenne pepper 2 tablespoons cornstarch	*4* In a bowl, combine the beans, rice, onion mixture, cilantro, garlic powder, cumin, chili powder, and cayenne pepper. In another bowl, combine the reserved black bean juice with the cornstarch to make a paste. Mix the paste into the black bean mixture.
¾ cup shredded cheddar cheese	*5* Spread the black bean mixture in the pie shell. Cover with the cheese. Bake for 15 to 20 minutes, until the cheese starts to brown. Let set for 15 minutes before serving.

Per serving: Kcalories 303 (From Fat 112); Fat 12g (Saturated 5g); Cholesterol 15mg; Sodium 435mg; Carbohydrate 37g (Dietary Fiber 5g); Protein 10g.

Tip: This recipe is a great way to get most of the basic food groups covered. The beans, peppers, and cilantro can stop a craving for Mexican food dead in its tracks. Serve it up with a crisp green salad to round out your meal plan.

Tip: When using canned anything, like beans or veggies, whenever possible, drain and rinse the food before cooking to get rid of excess sodium. But before you toss out the liquid, remember to double-check the recipe. Some recipes, like the one for Black Bean Pie here, use the liquid in the recipe.

Southwestern Hummus

Prep time: 10 min • **Yield:** 4 servings

Ingredients	Directions
1½ tablespoons minced garlic	**1** Place the garlic, beans, salsa, lime juice, cumin, chili powder, cayenne pepper, olive oil, cilantro, and salt and pepper to taste in a food processor. Adjust seasonings to taste. Place in a covered bowl. Chill in the refrigerator for 2 to 3 hours to allow flavors to meld, or blend thoroughly.
2 cans (15 ounces each) garbanzo beans, drained and rinsed	
¼ cup salsa	
2 tablespoons fresh lime juice	**2** When ready to serve, spread the hummus in the bottom of a medium-sized serving bowl, and top with the garnishes in the following order: light sour cream, avocado, cilantro, and black olives.
1 teaspoon cumin	
½ teaspoon chili powder	
1 teaspoon cayenne (more or less as you prefer)	
1 tablespoon olive oil	
⅓ cup roughly chopped cilantro	
Salt and pepper	
Garnishes (optional):	
1 tablespoon light sour cream	
2 tablespoons diced avocado	
1 tablespoon minced cilantro	
1 tablespoon minced black olives	

Per serving: Kcalories 170 (From Fat 48); Fat 5g (Saturated 1g); Cholesterol 0mg; Sodium 477mg; Carbohydrate 24g (Dietary Fiber 6g); Protein 7g.

Tip: This creamy spread (with little fat!) makes for a surprisingly healthy appetizer — great served with whole-wheat pita bread wedges, baked tortilla chips, or raw vegetables. (If you're looking for other delicious dipper ideas to pair with this tasty spread, check out Chapter 7.)

Gluten-Free Skillet Cornbread

Prep time: 15 min • **Cook time:** 25 min • **Yield:** 8 servings

Ingredients	Directions
2 eggs	**1** Place a skillet in the oven and preheat the oven to 400 degrees.
3 tablespoons sugar	
1 cup buttermilk	**2** In a medium bowl, beat the eggs and sugar. Stir in the buttermilk.
1½ cups stone-ground cornmeal	
¾ cup gluten-free flour	**3** In another medium bowl, combine and stir together the cornmeal, flour, baking soda, baking powder, and salt. Add the dry ingredients to the wet ingredients, and mix well.
¼ teaspoon baking soda	
2 teaspoons baking powder	
½ teaspoon salt	
2 tablespoons melted light butter	**4** Stir in the butter and applesauce.
2 tablespoons applesauce	**5** Remove the skillet from the oven and spray lightly with oil spray.
	6 Pour the batter into the skillet and place in the oven. Bake for 25 minutes, until a toothpick inserted into the center of the cornbread is clean and dry.
	7 Allow to cool before attempting to cut and serve.

Per serving: Kcalories 176 (From Fat 36); Fat 4g (Saturated 1g); Cholesterol 47mg; Sodium 74mg; Carbohydrate 32g (Dietary Fiber 5g); Protein 5g.

Vary It! You can experiment with other flavors if you want. Add some sliced jalapeños for a spicy taste, or add some thyme for a more savory taste.

Chapter 11

The Key Role of Vegetables

In This Chapter

▶ Giving old favorites a fresh taste

▶ Making "noodles" from firm vegetables

▶ Mixing up tasty mushroom dishes

▶ Dressing up vegetables for special occasions

▶ Enjoying vegetarian entrees

*O*ur bodies thrive on the fantastic phyto-chemicals, must-have vitamins and nutrients, and fabulous fiber found in vegetables, but most people don't eat enough of them. Yet there are so many ways you can eat them: in soups, in salads, puréed in sauces, on the side, or as the main event. Whether you eat them cooked or raw, using fresh or frozen products, you can improve your health today by increasing the amount of vegetables you eat.

In this chapter, we help you update common vegetables in exciting new ways. We focus on using mushrooms in delicious ways. We help you create some special-occasion recipes to impress your guests. And finally, we show you how to enjoy delicious vegetarian entrees.

Adding a New Twist to Old Favorites (and Not-So-Favorites)

Most people have a vegetable that has haunted them since childhood. Whether you had the misfortune to taste flavorless collard greens at a family reunion when you were 9 or were forced to sit in front of a plate of lukewarm boiled carrots you just couldn't choke down, you probably have one you just don't like. Well, hopefully, we're about to change that.

In this section, we give you delicious recipes using traditional vegetables that you can find in the kitchens of most people but that you may not be fond of — yet. But never fear — after trying a few, you'll have a whole new appreciation for them.

Including delicious extras

The following recipes focus on adding tasty flavors such as rice vinegar, herbs, and cheese to old standby vegetables like collard greens, broccoli, and zucchini. Try them the next time you want to add some zing to your veggies.

Broccoli with Creamy Lemon Sauce

Prep time: 10 min • **Cook time:** 35 min • **Yield:** 6 servings

Ingredients	Directions
⅔ cup lowfat cottage cheese	*1* In a blender, combine the cottage cheese, milk, Parmesan cheese, lemon juice, turmeric, and white pepper to taste and purée until the mixture achieves a thin consistency, about 30 seconds.
¼ cup evaporated skim milk	
2 tablespoons grated Parmesan cheese	
1 teaspoon lemon juice	*2* Heat the sauce in a skillet, stirring occasionally, until heated through, but do not boil.
⅛ teaspoon ground turmeric	
White pepper	*3* Serve the sauce over the warm broccoli.
3 cups hot cooked broccoli florets	

Per serving: Kcalories 45 (From Fat 8); Fat 1g (Saturated 1g); Cholesterol 3mg; Sodium 155mg; Carbohydrate 4g (Dietary Fiber 1g); Protein 6g.

Zucchini and Parmigiano-Reggiano Salad

Prep time: 15 min • **Yield:** 4 servings

Ingredients	Directions
3 medium zucchini, peeled and sliced ½ cup Parmigiano-Reggiano, shaved thin 1 tablespoon lemon juice 4 tablespoons extra-virgin olive oil 1 teaspoon sea salt ½ teaspoon pepper 2 tablespoons chopped lemon verbena	Place the zucchini in a bowl and shave the Parmigiano-Reggiano in the bowl. Add the lemon juice, olive oil, salt, pepper, and verbena. Toss to incorporate the ingredients and serve.

Per serving: Kcalories 188 (From Fat 151); Fat 17g (Saturated 4g); Cholesterol 8mg; Sodium 766mg; Carbohydrate 5g (Dietary Fiber 2g); Protein 6g.

Tip: Lemon verbena is a potent herb, with a strong lemon flavor. Look for it in specialty food markets. Alternatively, look for it at your local nursery and grow your own. If you can't find it, you can always pick another herb (like tarragon or basil). The substitution will change the flavor but will still be delicious.

Chunky Zucchini-Tomato Curry

Prep time: 10 min • **Cook time:** 20 min • **Yield:** 4 servings

Ingredients	Directions
2 tablespoons olive oil	**1** Heat the olive oil in a large nonstick skillet. Sauté the onion, ginger, and garlic for about 5 minutes, or until the onions are translucent. Add the coriander and curry powder. Continue cooking 1 minute.
1 medium red onion, finely diced	
2 teaspoons grated fresh ginger	
4 cloves garlic, minced	**2** Stir in the tomatoes and zucchini. Simmer approximately 10 minutes, or until the zucchini is tender.
1 teaspoon ground coriander	
2 teaspoons curry powder	
1 cup canned crushed tomatoes	
1 pound zucchini, quartered lengthwise and large diced	

Per serving: Kcalories 97 (From Fat 64); Fat 8g (Saturated 1g); Cholesterol 0mg; Sodium 38mg; Carbohydrate 8g (Dietary Fiber 3g); Protein 2g.

Enhancing natural flavors with dry steaming

Dry steaming refers to cooking vegetables in their own natural juices rather than adding additional moisture. In the case of carrots, they have a medium to high moisture content, so when you heat them in a closed environment (like in a pot with a tight-fitting lid), they use the liquid that they give off during the cooking process to create steam and facilitate the cooking process. So the food is essentially steamed without adding any water. You get a similar effect when you microwave vegetables without adding water.

Don't microwave vegetables, or anything else, in a completely closed container. Always provide a vent of some sort for steam to escape.

Dry-Steamed Dilled Carrots

Prep time: 10 min • **Cook time:** 35–40 min • **Yield:** 12 servings

Ingredients	Directions
2 tablespoons butter 1 pound baby carrots ¼ cup minced fresh dill Salt and pepper	*1* Melt the butter in a deep skillet with a tight-fitting lid. Add the carrots. Cook over medium to medium-low heat for approximately 35 to 40 minutes. Shake the skillet occasionally during cooking, without removing the lid. *2* Remove the lid after 35 to 40 minutes and check to confirm that carrots are tender. Allow any excess moisture to evaporate from the skillet. Toss the carrots with the dill. Salt and pepper to taste.

Per serving: Kcalories 31 (From Fat 19); Fat 2g (Saturated 1g); Cholesterol 5mg; Sodium 62mg; Carbohydrate 3g (Dietary Fiber 1g); Protein 0g.

Gigante Beans

Prep time: 30 min plus overnight soaking • **Cook time:** 2 hr 20 min • **Yield:** 4 servings

Ingredients	Directions
9 ounces gigante beans, soaked overnight	**1** Drain the soaked beans and place them in a large pot.
¼ cup Greek olive oil	**2** Cover the beans well with water and bring to a boil for 10 minutes. Soak in the hot liquid for 10 more minutes.
½ red onion, finely diced	
1 garlic clove, finely sliced	**3** In a pot, heat the oil. Add the onion and cook on low for 3 minutes.
½ cup carrots, finely chopped	
½ cup celery, finely chopped	**4** Add the beans, garlic, carrots, celery, oregano, thyme, and tomato paste. Stir over a low heat for 3 minutes. Pour the contents into a bowl.
½ tablespoon dry Greek oregano	
½ tablespoon fresh thyme, finely chopped	**5** Add the vinegar to the hot pot, allow it to boil, and scrape the bottom of the pot. Return the contents to the pot.
½ tablespoon tomato paste	
⅓ cup sherry vinegar	
2 cups chopped tomatoes	**6** Add the tomatoes and water and bring to a boil.
1⅓ cups water	
Salt to taste	**7** Cover well with aluminum foil and bake for 2 hours at 300 degrees.
1 lemon, cut into wedges, for garnish	
¼ bunch Italian parsley, roughly chopped	**8** Season with salt and garnish with lemon wedges and parsley.

Per serving: Kcalories 171 (From Fat 45); Fat 5g (Saturated Fat 0g); Cholesterol 0mg; Sodium 40mg; Carbohydrate 30g (Dietary Fiber 9g); Protein 10g.

Note: Gigante is the Greek word for "giant." The type of bean used in this recipe is usually the Greek *fasolia gigandes* (giant white bean). The bean can be found at Mediterranean stores or specialty food markets. You can also use dried lima beans or dried Great Northern beans instead. The dish can be an appetizer, but it's often used as a main dish with whole-grain bread, olives, and raw scallions.

Blanching vegetables for optimum taste and nutrition

Blanching is a terrific technique for cooking vegetables without losing many of the vitamins that make them so healthy for you. It's also surprisingly simple. You immerse vegetables in boiling water, leave them in the water for a short period of time, and then *shock* them, or immerse them in ice-cold water to stop the cooking. This technique helps to prevent the vegetables from getting mushy.

Here are the detailed steps to follow for blanching vegetables.

1. **Bring salted water to vigorous boil in a 2-quart saucepan.**

2. **While the water is working up to a boil, prepare the ice bath.**

   Fill a medium-sized mixing bowl one-half to three-fourths full with ice. Add water to just cover the ice.

3. **Blanch the vegetables.**

   Place the trimmed vegetables, in batches if necessary, in the boiling water. Cook the vegetables until they're crisp tender.

   You want to keep a constant boil, but adding too many veggies at a time can slow down the process.

4. **Shock the vegetables.**

   Remove the vegetables with a slotted spoon and immediately place them in the ice bath. Remove them from the ice bath after the vegetables are completely cooled, usually 1 to 2 minutes.

   To check for doneness, remove a single vegetable piece with a slotted spoon; submerge it in the ice bath until it's cool enough to place in your mouth. Then actually taste it to check the texture. Do this step quickly so that if the veggies are ready, the rest of them in the boiling water won't overcook while you're testing.

5. **Reheat the vegetables and season as desired.**

Blanching times vary based on the vegetable and the size of the pieces, but check out Table 11-1 for approximate times for reference.

Table 11-1	Approximate Blanching Times for Vegetables	
Vegetable	**Size**	**Approximate Time**
Asparagus	Spears	3 to 4 minutes
Broccoli	Florets, bite sized	3 minutes
Brussels sprouts	Whole	3 to 5 minutes
Cabbage	Leaves	5 to 10 minutes
Carrots, baby	Whole	5 minutes
Carrots	Diced or strips	2 minutes
Cauliflower	Florets, bite sized	3 minutes
Corn	Cob	4 minutes
Eggplant	Slices	3 minutes
Green beans	Whole	3 minutes
Greens like spinach	Leaves	2 minutes
Mushrooms	Whole or caps	5 minutes
Okra	Pod	3 to 5 minutes
Peas, shelled	Whole	1½ minutes
Peas	Pod	2 to 3 minutes
Summer squash	Bite-sized chunks	3 minutes
Tomatoes	Whole, for peeling	1 minute
Zucchini	Bite-sized chunks	3 minutes

Haricot Vert

Prep time: 10 min • **Cook time:** 10 min • **Yield:** 6 servings

Ingredients	Directions
6 cups string beans **2 tablespoons butter** **Salt and pepper**	Cut off the ends of the beans and blanch in boiling water for 1 minute (see the instructions earlier in this section); remove and place them in a cold water bath with ice. Drain and reheat in a skillet with the butter and salt and pepper to taste.

Tip: Serve these tasty veggies with Veal Tenderloin with Chanterelle Mushrooms in Chapter 14.

Per serving: Kcalories 71 (From Fat 37); Fat 4g (Saturated 2g); Cholesterol 10mg; Sodium 101mg; Carbohydrate 9g (Dietary Fiber 4g); Protein 2g.

Note: Haricot vert (pronounced ah-ree-co VEHR) is a fancy French word that literally means "green beans" and refers to (surprise!) green beans, or what we sometimes call string beans. If you find true French haricot vert in a gourmet market, use them in this recipe. They're a bit smaller and thinner than common string beans, but the flavor is very similar. But if you can't find them, feel free to substitute fresh string beans. Canned beans won't work because they're already cooked beyond tender.

Using Vegetables in Place of Pasta

Pasta gets a lot of bad press these days, but the biggest problem with it is the portion size that most people typically eat. For healthy ways to include pasta and other grains in your diabetic diet, check out Chapter 10.

When you're craving the rich delicious Italian sauces but don't want the carbs of traditional pasta, veggies make a terrific substitute. Make "noodles" from strings of cucumber or slices of zucchini. Get started with this great Zucchini and Cucumber Linguine with Clams.

A *mandoline* is a handy tool to have around your kitchen. Take a look at it in Figure 11-1. It's a manual slicing device that quickly makes consistently sized cuts of foods. You can use it to julienne or make even ¼-inch strips of cucumber (as in the next recipe). You can make paper-thin strips of sweet potatoes for making your own baked chips or thick lemon wheels for water. Consider getting one to ease the prep work of making your own veggie noodles. Look for a mandoline at your local cooking supply store or gourmet shop.

Figure 11-1:
A mandoline makes quick work of slicing and creating juli-enne cuts.

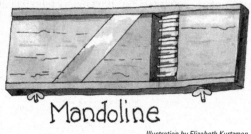

Mandoline

Illustration by Elizabeth Kurtzman

Zucchini and Cucumber Linguine with Clams

Prep time: 20 min • **Cook time:** 20 min • **Yield:** 4 servings

Ingredients	Directions
2 tablespoons olive oil	**1** Heat the olive oil in a sauté pan. Add the garlic, shallots, and red peppers and sauté until golden, approximately 10 minutes. Add the clams, white wine, and lemon juice. Cover and bring to a boil. Continue to cook until the clams open, approximately 5 minutes.
2 tablespoons chopped garlic	
2 tablespoons chopped shallots	
¼ cup minced red peppers	
18 to 24 Manila or littleneck clams	**2** When the clams open, add the butter, salt and pepper to taste, and the red pepper flakes. Remove the clams. Toss in the cucumber and zucchini noodles and heat until they are warm and wilted, approximately 7 minutes.
1½ cups white wine	
2 lemons (juice and zest)	
1 tablespoon butter	**3** Divide among 4 bowls and top each with the clams and the remaining juice. Garnish with the chopped parsley and lemon zest.
Salt and pepper	
1 teaspoon red pepper flakes	
1 large seedless cucumber, cut into long julienne strips to resemble noodles (use a mandoline or a sharp knife)	
1 large zucchini, julienned	
¼ cup chopped parsley	

Per serving: Kcalories 171 (From Fat 95); Fat 11g (Saturated 3g); Cholesterol 28mg; Sodium 188mg; Carbohydrate 10g (Dietary Fiber 3g); Protein 11g.

Tip: When purchasing clams and other shellfish, be sure the shells are closed. The open ones can be contaminated and cause severe food-borne illness.

Making the Most of Mushrooms

If you haven't taken a tour of the produce department lately, you might be surprised by the variety of mushrooms out there (some can be seen in Figure 11-2), each with a distinct look and flavor. In this section, chefs from several award-winning vegetarian restaurants have supplied some creative ways to get the most flavor out of their favorite fungi. And don't forget that mushrooms have many health benefits especially improved nutrition with increased vitamins B and D and lots of minerals.

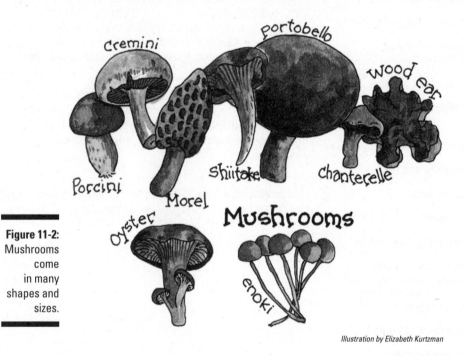

Figure 11-2:
Mushrooms come in many shapes and sizes.

Illustration by Elizabeth Kurtzman

Portobello Mushroom Sandwich

Prep time: 10 min • **Cook time:** 5 min • **Yield:** 4 servings

Ingredients	*Directions*
4 medium-sized portobello mushrooms **8 tablespoons extra-virgin olive oil** **Salt and pepper to taste** **Chopped fresh herbs such as thyme, parsley, or chives** **8 pieces whole-grain bread, toasted**	*1* With a brush or damp cloth, remove any dirt from the mushrooms. Remove the stem and save for another use. Place the mushrooms in a wide bowl and coat on all sides with the olive oil. Sprinkle generously with salt and pepper and the chopped fresh herbs.
	2 Preheat a broiler, or start a charcoal fire. When hot, place the mushrooms on the grill over the fire. Grill for about 1 minute on each side. The mushrooms should be juicy but not shrunken.
	3 Cut the buns in half lengthwise or cut the bread to look like hamburger buns. Place the grilled mushrooms on the buns and serve warm.

Per serving: Kcalories 397 (Calories from Fat 261); Fat 29g (Saturated 4g); Cholesterol 0mg; Sodium 406g; Carbohydrate 29g (Dietary Fiber 5g); Protein 7g.

Tip: Look for 100 percent whole-wheat hamburger buns to make this dish even easier to prepare.

Mushroom Garlic Medley

Prep time: 15 min • **Cook time:** 15 min • **Yield:** 6 servings

Ingredients	Directions
¼ cup abalone mushrooms (sliced thinly)	**1** Blanch the mushrooms and vegetables (except for the Enoki mushrooms). Take a look at the section "Blanching vegetables for optimum taste and nutrition," earlier in this chapter for help. Drain well. Set aside.
½ cup oyster mushrooms (sliced thinly)	
1½ cups shiitake mushrooms (sliced thinly)	
2½ cups button mushrooms (sliced thinly)	**2** In a wok, heat olive oil over medium-high heat and sauté the sliced garlic until golden brown. Add blanched mushrooms and vegetables, and Sweet and Savory Sauce (see the next recipe) to the wok and sauté together with the garlic for 4 to 5 minutes.
1 cup broccoli (separate the individual heads)	
¼ cup carrots (sliced thinly)	
½ cup zucchini (sliced thinly)	**3** Meanwhile, separate the enoki mushrooms into separate stalks. Cut the base of each mushroom bunch and then pull each stalk to separate it. Set aside.
⅓ cup snow peas	
¼ cup red bell pepper (sliced into long strips)	**4** Place the mushroom mixture in a heated serving dish. Garnish with enoki mushrooms.
¼ cup green bell pepper (sliced into long strips)	
⅓ cup garlic (sliced thinly)	
1 tablespoon olive oil	
¼ cup enoki mushrooms	

Sweet and Savory Sauce

½ cup pears (diced)

½ cup apples (diced)

½ cup oranges (diced)

¼ cup onions (diced)

¼ cup radishes (diced)

2 tablespoons ginger paste

2 tablespoons sesame seed

½ cup plus 3 tablespoons water, divided

3 ounces sake

1 tablespoon agave nectar

½ tablespoon sesame oil

1½ teaspoons mushroom powder (available at spice stores or online)

½ tablespoon reduced-sodium soy sauce

1 teaspoon black pepper

1 tablespoon potato powder (available at spice stores or online)

1 Combine diced pears, apples, oranges, onions, radishes, ginger paste, sesame seeds, and ½ cup water in a mixer. Mix on low speed until mixture blended.

2 Place mixture into a pot. Add sake, agave nectar, sesame oil, mushroom powder, soy sauce, and black pepper.

3 In a separate bowl, mix potato powder with 3 tablespoons water. Add the potato powder mixture to the pot. Let the sauce simmer for 5 minutes over low flame, stirring continuously.

Per serving: Kcalories 128 (Calories from Fat 47); Fat 5g (Saturated 1g); Cholesterol 10mg; Sodium 61mg; Carbohydrate 19g (Dietary Fiber 4g); Protein 4g.

Organic Tofu and Shiitake Mushrooms

Prep time: 30 min • **Cook time:** 3 min • **Yield:** 4 servings

Ingredients	Directions
24 ounces organic firm tofu	*1* Cut tofu into rectangles with approximate dimensions of 3½ inches by 4 inches with ½-inch thickness. Coat the pieces with soybean powder.
¼ cup organic soybean powder	
1 tablespoon olive oil	*2* Over medium-high heat, heat olive oil in a sauté pan. Fry the tofu with olive oil until the pieces are golden brown.
12 pieces medium-size fresh shiitake mushrooms	
Vegetarian Oyster Sauce	*3* Meanwhile, in a separate pan, pan-fry the shiitake mushrooms. Set aside.
2½ ounces vegetarian oyster sauce	
2 tablespoons agave nectar	*4* Mix all the ingredients for the sauce in a pot and heat for about 2 minutes over low flame.
1 tablespoon water	
1 teaspoon tomato ketchup	*5* Put a piece of shiitake mushroom on top of each of the tofu pieces. Pour the sauce over the tofu and shiitake mushrooms and serve.
1 teaspoon sesame seeds	
½ teaspoon sesame oil	
Dash of black pepper	
2 sesame leaves (chopped into small pieces), basil leaves can be used if sesame leaves are not available	

Per serving: Kcalories 344 (Calories from Fat 144); Fat 16g (Saturated 2g); Cholesterol 0mg; Sodium 490mg; Carbohydrate 22g (Dietary Fiber 7g); Protein 36g.

Tip: You can find the more exotic ingredients (like the soybean powder, vegetarian oyster sauce, and agave nectar) at your local natural food store.

Giving Veggies the Gourmet Treatment

Vegetables are ripe for dressing up with the full gourmet treatment. They're flavorful on their own, but they take most seasonings, spices, and cooking techniques very well. You really can't mess them up unless you overcook them. Experiment with your favorite recipes by using the techniques in this chapter. Also, try a few that you haven't tried before just to broaden your vegetable horizon.

Pickled Vegetables

Prep time: 30 min • **Cook time:** 3 min • **Yield:** 20 servings

Ingredients	Directions
1 tablespoon yellow mustard seed	**1** Combine the mustard seed, fennel seed, peppercorns, pepperoncini, bay leaves, water, vinegar, thyme, sugar, and salt in a large pot and bring to a boil. Add the vegetables and simmer for about 3 minutes.
1 teaspoon fennel seed	
1 teaspoon black peppercorns	
4 dried pepperoncini	**2** Turn off the heat, but leave the vegetables in the pickling solution. The residual heat will cook them through.
2 bay leaves	
3 cups water	**3** Discard the pickling juice and store in the refrigerator for up to 5 days.
1 cup white wine vinegar	
3 sprigs thyme	
1 cup sugar	
3 tablespoons salt	
3 pounds vegetables (such as carrots, cauliflower, cherry peppers, fennel, onions, or turnips), cleaned and cut into bite-sized pieces	

Tip: Serve these pickles with sandwiches or fried fish or just snack on them on their own.

Per serving: Kcalories 28 (From Fat 0); Fat 0g (Saturated 0g); Cholesterol 0mg; Sodium 283mg; Carbohydrate 7g (Dietary Fiber 2g); Protein 1g.

Asian Vegetable Stir-Fry

Prep time: 40 min • **Cook time:** 20 min • **Yield:** 4 servings

Ingredients	Directions
2 ounces dehydrated wild mushrooms	*1* Place the mushrooms in a heatproof bowl and cover them with the boiling water. Allow them to reconstitute for 30 minutes. Remove the mushrooms from the water. Chop them and reserve. Strain the liquid through a coffee filter to remove the grit. Combine the mushroom liquid, soy sauce, garlic, and gingerroot. Set aside.
¼ cup boiling water	
1 tablespoon light soy sauce	
2 cloves garlic, minced	
1½ teaspoons grated fresh gingerroot	*2* Heat the oil in a wok or nonstick skillet. Stir-fry the mushrooms, bok choy, red bell pepper, carrots, and broccoli for 3 minutes. Add the soy sauce mixture and snow peas. Reduce the heat and continue cooking until the veggies are crisp tender and the sauce thickens.
2 tablespoons canola oil	
2 cups baby bok choy, sliced in half	
1 red bell pepper, seeded and julienned	
½ carrot, thinly sliced on the diagonal	
1 cup broccoli florets	
1 cup snow peas, trimmed	

Per serving: Kcalories 137 (From Fat 66); Fat 7g (Saturated 1g); Cholesterol 0mg; Sodium 176mg; Carbohydrate 17g (Dietary Fiber 4g); Protein 4g.

Tip: With this stir-fry, be creative and use any vegetables that you like. The health benefits here don't get any better! All these vegetables in combination are rich in countless vitamins and minerals, notably vitamins A, C, B6, folate, calcium, and potassium. This stir-fry is prepared with minimal oil, so it remains quite low in total fat and calories. It's also rich in fiber, which makes it great for weight management, heart health, and especially blood sugar control. If you like, round out this dish with some tofu or chicken to get a bit of lean protein, and serve over a bed of brown rice for some more fiber, as well.

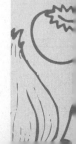

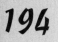

Goat-Cheese-Stuffed Zucchini with Yellow Tomato Sauce

Prep time: 40 min • **Cook time:** 25–30 min • **Yield:** 6 servings

Ingredients	Directions
6 medium green zucchini **1 pound goat cheese (room temperature)** **¼ cup bread crumbs** **Zest of 1 lemon** **¼ cup basil chiffonade (see the tip at the end of this recipe)** **Salt and pepper** **1 tablespoon olive oil**	*1* Preheat the oven to 350 degrees. Wash the zucchini and pat dry. Cut the ends off the zucchini and then cut each zucchini in half to create 2 pieces of equal length. Use a paring knife or melon baller to core out the center of the zucchini. *2* Put the goat cheese in a bowl and add the bread crumbs, lemon zest, and basil. Season with salt and pepper to taste. Mix well and taste for seasoning. Spoon the cheese mixture into the zucchini shells. *3* Drizzle the olive oil on the zucchini, season with salt and pepper to taste, and place on a baking sheet. Bake until the cheese begins to bubble and the bread crumbs start to brown, about 30 minutes. *4* Remove the zucchini from the oven, drizzle the Yellow Tomato Sauce (see the next recipe) on top of them, and return to the oven for 1 to 2 minutes.

Tip: Chiffonade literally means "made of rags," and it pretty well describes what the final product looks like. Leafy lettuce or herbs are rolled together tightly and then thinly sliced width-wise to form long, stringy strips.

Yellow Tomato Sauce

4 ripened yellow tomatoes (substitute red tomatoes if yellow ones aren't available)

¼ cup minced garlic

2 tablespoons olive oil

Salt and pepper

1 Core the tomatoes, blanch in salted water for 10 seconds, and then shock in an ice water bath. (See "Blanching vegetables for optimum taste and nutrition," earlier in this chapter, for instructions.) Allow the tomatoes to chill for a few minutes and then remove from the water and peel the skin. Cut the tomatoes in half and squeeze out the pulp and seeds.

2 Place the tomatoes in a blender, add the garlic, and blend. With the blender on high, drizzle in the olive oil until the sauce achieves a smooth, even consistency, approximately 3 to 5 minutes. Season with salt and pepper to taste.

Per serving: Kcalories 411 (From Fat 272); Fat 30g (Saturated 17g); Cholesterol 60mg; Sodium 661mg; Carbohydrate 17g (Dietary Fiber 4g); Protein 21g.

Tip: This vibrant dish is high in protein and quite low in carbohydrate, making it suitable for people managing their blood sugars. Keep in mind, however, that goat cheese is quite rich and high in saturated fat. Be sure to enjoy these zucchinis in moderation.

Vegetable Fritto Misto

Prep time: 30 min • **Cook time:** 35 min • **Yield:** 4 servings

Ingredients	Directions
4 tablespoons canola oil	**1** Heat the oil in a deep skillet until it starts smoking. While you're waiting for the oil to heat, place the artichoke hearts, cauliflower, olives, and mushrooms in the milk in a shallow bowl and soak. Place the soaked veggies in a resealable plastic bag with the flour. Shake to coat the veggies with flour. Put the floured vegetables into a strainer and shake off the excess flour.
½ cup artichoke hearts	
½ head cauliflower, chopped into florets	
10 pitted green olives	
1 large portobello mushroom, large dice	**2** Carefully place the vegetables in batches into the hot oil. Fry for 3 to 5 minutes, or until golden brown.
2 cups lowfat milk	
2 cups flour	**3** Remove the vegetables from the oil onto paper towels and season lightly with salt and pepper. Place them in a bowl and serve with a wedge or two of lemon, if desired.
Salt and pepper	
Lemon wedges (optional)	

Per serving: Kcalories 192 (From Fat 90); Fat 10g (Saturated 1g); Cholesterol 1mg; Sodium 480mg; Carbohydrate 22g (Dietary Fiber 3g); Protein 5g.

Tip: To ensure that your food absorbs the least amount of oil possible, make sure the oil is very hot before you begin frying it. This step ensures that your food gets a quick, crispy outer coating without getting saturated in oil. When the veggies are finished, drain them well on paper towels to get rid of some of the excess oil.

Note: Moderation is the key when enjoying any fried foods. Many diabetics are encouraged to stay away from fried food entirely. In general, it's good advice because so many foods are heavily battered with starchy concoctions that no one needs to eat. But on occasion, you can enjoy fried foods that are lightly *dredged,* or lightly coated, in flour, as in this recipe.

Expanding Your Meal Options with Vegetarian Entrees

When you hear the word "vegetarian," you might think bland tofu or piles of raw vegetables. But vegetarian cuisine is undergoing a true renaissance, as new vegan and vegetarian restaurants open in cities large and small. More people are choosing to eat vegetarian meals as part of their regular diets. Vegetarian meals can be part of a healthy diabetic diet.

Vietnamese-Style Stuffed Grape Leaves

Prep time: 17 min • **Cook time:** 15 min • **Yield:** 6 servings

Ingredients	Directions
2 cups thinly sliced fresh shii-take mushrooms	**1** Heat a nonstick sauté pan over medium heat, add the shiitakes, ginger, garlic, black beans, and vegetable stock. Cook the mushrooms until soft and most of the stock evaporates. Add the tofu, rice, and cilantro. Cook the mixture, stirring until heated through. Season mixture with Tamari (or salt if using) and black pepper. Set aside.
2 teaspoons minced ginger	
2 cloves garlic, minced	
1 tablespoon Chinese fermented black soybeans, minced	
⅓ cup vegetable stock	
1½ cups crumbled firm tofu	**2** Place a grape leaf on a flat work surface. Place 1 heaping tablespoon of filling in the center of the leaf, then fold up the leaf like a spring roll or burrito. Repeat with 2 more rolls and then skewer 3 together. Repeat with remaining grape leaves and skewers.
1½ cups cooked brown rice	
4 tablespoons cilantro leaves	
1 tablespoon Tamari or salt to taste	
Black pepper to taste	**3** Place the skewers on a sheet pan and lightly brush with plum sauce (see the next recipe). Sprinkle with sesame seeds. Broil for 2 minutes until heated through and the sauce caramelizes on top.
6 wooden skewers, soaked in water	
18 brined large grape leaves, rinsed and dried	
1 tablespoon sesame seeds	**4** Serve 1 skewer per person with 3 lettuce leaves, and a sprig of cilantro, basil, and mint with 3 tablespoons of the sauce in a small bowl or on the plate.
18 Romaine or butter lettuce leaves	
1 bunch cilantro	
1 bunch mint	
1 bunch Thai basil	

Sweet and Spicy Plum – Miso Sauce

2 ripe red-fleshed plums, seed removed, diced

1 clove garlic peeled

1 tablespoon minced ginger

1 Thai chile

2 tablespoons agave nectar

1 tablespoon rice vinegar

4 tablespoons white or chick-pea miso

½ cup water

Place all ingredients in a blender and blend until smooth. Adjust the sweetener and vinegar to taste.

Per serving: Kcalories 252 (Calories from Fat 64); Fat 5g (Saturated 7g); Cholesterol 0mg; Sodium 851mg; Carbohydrate 37g (Dietary Fiber 5g); Protein 14g.

Asparagus Pizza with Fontina and Truffle Oil

Prep time: 45 min plus 90 min for rising • **Cook time:** 20 min • **Yield:** 6 servings

Ingredients	Directions
1 package dry active yeast	*1* To make the dough, dissolve the yeast in the ½ cup water in a small warmed bowl. Stir in ½ cup white flour, cover, and let rest for 10 to 15 minutes until bubbles form on the surface.
½ cup warm water (110 to 115 degrees)	
1 to 2 cups white flour	
1 cup whole wheat flour	*2* Meanwhile, in a larger bowl, mix ½ cup of white flour, whole-wheat flour, and rye flour, and 1½ teaspoons salt. Make a well in the center and add the yeast mixture and the remaining warm water and olive oil. Mix well and knead until the dough is smooth, adding more flour if necessary. Place the dough in a lightly oiled bowl and turn over in order to coat the top of the dough. Cover and put in a warm place for at least 1½ hours.
3 tablespoons rye flour	
1 teaspoon salt, divided	
⅔ cup warm water	
2 tablespoons olive oil	
1 pound fresh asparagus	
Cornmeal as needed	*3* Bring a medium size pan of water to a boil over high heat, and cut the asparagus into ¼-inch slices, discarding the tough stems. Blanch and shock the asparagus. For details on how to blanch and shock vegetables, take a look at the section, "Blanching vegetables for optimum taste and nutrition," earlier in this chapter. Set the asparagus aside until ready to use.
1 cup fontina, or Monterey Jack cheese, grated	
¼ cup good quality Parmesan, grated	
½ tablespoon white truffle oil	
	4 Place a large baking stone on the bottom shelf of an oven. Preheat the oven to 500 degrees 30 minutes before baking.

5 Punch down the dough and place on a lightly floured wooden board or counter. Cut into 6 equal pieces. Cover the dough you are not working with a bowl or a dry towel. With your hands, shape one of the pieces of dough into a round disc. Then roll it flatter with a rolling pin. Place this on a *pizza peel* (a large paddle with a long handle used to transfer a raw pizza to the oven) covered with 1 tablespoon cornmeal, and stretch into a thin round with your fingers. Make sure the pizza dough can slide, and isn't stuck to the pizza peel. Cover the dough with the fontina cheese, then the asparagus, then the Parmesan. Repeat with remaining pieces of dough.

6 Place pizza in the oven and bake for 15 to 20 minutes until it is lightly browned on the bottom. Remove from the oven and sprinkle with the truffle oil and serve.

Per serving: Kcalories 265 (Calories from Fat 116); Fat 13g (Saturated 5g); Cholesterol 24mg; Sodium 600mg; Carbohydrate 28g (Dietary Fiber 4g); Protein 12g.

Tip: The pizza dough will remain usable at least all day if kept cool, and more if refrigerated after the first rising. If you do refrigerate the dough, allow at least 1 hour for it to come to room temperature.

Baby Artichokes, Gigante Beans, and Summer Vegetable Cartoccio with Creamy Polenta

Prep time: 45 min • **Cook time:** 30 min • **Yield:** 6 servings

Ingredients	Directions
1 quart of water	*1* Preheat the oven to 400 degrees.
1 head of garlic, cloves peeled or 18 medium to large garlic cloves	*2* Blanch the garlic cloves in 1 quart of water for 1 minute; then drain and set aside. Add the lemon juice to the boiling water. Clean the artichokes, and cut them in half. Blanch until the heart of the artichoke is just soft. Drain and reserve.
Juice from ½ lemon	
6 baby to mid-size artichokes	
6 pieces of bakers parchment or foil cut into 8- to 10-inch squares	*3* Place 1 piece of parchment (or foil if using) on a flat surface. Place 2 artichoke halves in the center, followed by 3 cloves of garlic, ¼ cup of the beans, 2 oyster mushrooms, 2 pieces of tomato, some of the summer squash, plus any other vegetable you are using. Top with basil leaves, rosemary sprig, a slice of lemon, a few capers, salt, pepper, and chile flakes if using. Pour 2 tablespoons of the stock or wine over the ingredients. Fold the parchment over the filling, and crimp the edges until sealed. Place sealed packet on a baking pan. Repeat with remaining parchment and ingredients.
1½ cup of cooked gigante beans, or canellini beans	
12 oyster mushrooms	
3 ripe Roma or other tomato, quartered	
2 summer squash, diced	
Other vegetables of choice	
½ bunch basil, leaves picked	*4* Bake for 15 minutes. Place the baked cartoccio in a large shallow bowl with a portion of the Creamy Polenta (see the next recipe) and present to your guests.
6 small sprigs of rosemary	
1 lemon sliced into 6 slices	
1 tablespoon capers	
Salt, pepper, and chile flakes to taste	
1 cup vegetable stock or white wine	

Creamy Polenta

1½ cups polenta

6 cups vegetables stock or water

1 tablespoon nutritional yeast

Salt and pepper to taste

1 Heat the stock or water in a saucepan to boiling. Whisk in the polenta, turn down the heat to a simmer and continue whisking for 2 minutes. Cook the polenta, whisking often for 20 minutes or until the polenta pulls away from the side of the pan and the grains are soft.

2 Whisk in the nutritional yeast and adjust salt and pepper to taste. Remove from heat and reserve. Set aside. When reheating, add more water to thin if needed.

Per serving: Kcalories 446 (Calories from Fat 26); Fat 0g (Saturated 0); Cholesterol 0mg; Sodium 1,000mg; Carbohydrate 93g (Dietary Fiber 24g); Protein 28g.

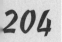

Asparagus Bread Pudding Layered with Fontina

Prep time: 45 min • **Cook time:** 60 min • **Yield:** 4 servings

Ingredients	Directions
Non-stick cooking spray 6 to 8 thick slices whole-grain bread, dry 1½ to 2 cups nonfat milk 2 pounds asparagus 2 eggs 1 teaspoon salt 2 teaspoons freshly ground black pepper 2 tablespoons freshly grated Parmesan cheese ½ cup Fontina cheese, Swiss cheese or other white cheese, shredded	**1** Preheat oven to 350 degrees. Spray a 2-quart soufflé dish with non-stick cooking spray; set aside. **2** Place the bread in a single layer in a shallow dish. Pour 1½ cups milk over the bread. Let the bread soak until the bread has absorbed the milk and becomes soft, about 30 minutes. Press the bread slices to extract the milk. Measure the milk; you should be able to squeeze ½ cup milk from the bread. If not, make up the difference with the additional ½ cup milk as needed. Set the milk and bread aside. **3** Meanwhile, trim the asparagus, removing the woody ends. Cut the remaining stalks on the diagonal into thin slivers each about 2 inches long and ⅜ of an inch thick. Blanch slivered asparagus until barely tender. Shock the blanched asparagus immediately. Drain and set aside. **4** In a bowl, beat together the eggs, salt, pepper, and the ½ cup milk from the bread soaking until well blended. Layer ⅓ of the bread in the prepared dish. Set 6 or 8 asparagus slivers aside and top the bread layer with half of the remaining asparagus. Spread ⅓ of each of the cheeses over the asparagus. **5** Repeat the layers, using half of the remaining bread, all of the remaining asparagus, and half of the remaining cheese. Arrange the remaining bread on top, spread the remaining cheese over it, and garnish with the reserved asparagus slivers. Pour the milk-egg mixture over the layers. **6** Bake in the preheated oven until the top is golden brown and a knife inserted in the middle of the pudding comes out clean, about 45 minutes.

Per serving: Kcalories 260 (Calories from Fat 86); Fat 10g (Saturated 4g); Cholesterol 126mg; Sodium 1,018mg; Carbohydrate 29g (Dietary Fiber 5g); Protein 18g.

Chapter 12

Fish: Good Protein, Good Fat

In This Chapter

▶ Investigating the health benefits of seafood

▶ Trying your hand at different fish preparation methods

▶ Including shellfish in your diet

Seafood is a great protein source, especially for diabetics. It has lower saturated fat, cholesterol, and carbohydrates than any other protein source. Much of it has a mild flavor that takes on the flavor of its accompanying ingredients and preparation methods, so you can have an almost endless variety of flavors and dishes. It cooks up quickly, so it can be ready when you are.

In this chapter, we convince you (in case you need it) that seafood is an excellent food choice to include in a diabetic diet. We give you plenty of recipes and fun new ways to prepare all kinds of fish dishes. And finally, we give you tips for preparing shellfish.

Identifying Good Reasons to Serve Seafood

Like meat and poultry, seafood supplies high-quality protein, balancing the fats and carbohydrates in the meal and providing calories that have little effect on blood glucose. But the benefits of eating fish extend beyond this:

✔ The oceans are a rich reservoir of minerals, and all creatures that live in the sea are in part made of these minerals. When you eat fish, you are likely also to be consuming iodine, selenium, phosphorus, potassium, iron, and calcium.

✔ Eating seafood regularly may help improve kidney function in patients with severe diabetes.

✔ Seafood is a good source of B vitamins, especially niacin, and also contains fat-soluble vitamin A. In addition, fatty fish are one of the few food sources of vitamin D.

✔ The most important nutrient in fish may well be the omega-3 fatty acids. These polyunsaturated fatty acids are especially high in the fat and oils of fish that live in cold water. (Because these oils stay liquid at room temperature, they may help insulate the fish against the cold.) The omega-3 fatty acids appear to lower the undesirable form of cholesterol, LDL cholesterol, and to raise the desirable form, HDL cholesterol. These fats also have an anti-inflammatory effect. The fish with the highest percentage of these healthy oils are salmon, sardines, tuna, and mackerel.

Healthy Americans are encouraged to eat two seafood servings per week on a regular basis.

Preparing Fish in Healthy Ways

You don't need to deep-fry your catch of the day or order deep-fried fish when you eat out in order to get fish that tastes good. Not only is this type of fish loaded with fat, but the type of fat is usually unhealthy. When fats heat to high temperatures, such as in deep-frying, toxic by-products are formed. It is far better to eat seafood prepared by methods such as baking, pan roasting, or grilling — all delicious and healthy ways of cooking fish. You can use a variety of methods to cook fish the healthy way:

✔ **Baking:** Baking is one of the first techniques most people learn when they're learning to cook. In fact, many people don't "learn" to bake; they simply seem to know how to bake. Technically speaking, *baking* means to cook something by surrounding it with dry heat. In most cases, you bake in an oven, a closed environment where you control the temperature.

✔ **Poaching:** Poaching is a method of cooking that gently cooks the food in a small amount of liquid, just below the boiling point. In the case of seafood, this liquid is often highly flavored with herbs, wine, stock, and other seasonings.

✔ **Pan roasting:** In the strictest culinary terms, *pan roasting* is a two-step process that first sears and seals a thicker piece of meat or chicken in a pan on the stovetop and then finishes that piece in the oven, in the same pan you started in. So, when we're talking about seafood, the term *pan roasting* is probably not exactly accurate. Because seafood cooks so fast, there's usually not a need to finish it in the oven. But you can make a terrific sauce in the same pan you seared your fish in.

Use a quality sauté pan that heats evenly. And make sure to heat it up well before you place your fish in to ensure an even, quick crust.

✔ **Grilling:** Grilling is similar to broiling, but the heat comes from a different direction. In grilling, the heat source is under the food. In broiling, the heat source is above the food.

Tuna is an excellent fish for grilling. Its meat is firm, not flaky like white fish. It stands up nicely to spices and flavorings. And because it's usually served extremely rare, it takes very little time to cook.

We start off this section with a soup. Fish soup is a found on all menus of restaurants close to the sea. Common names for fish soup or fish stew include bisque, bouillabaisse, chowder, and cioppino. Whatever fish happens to be available at the time goes into the soup, so the taste changes — but it's always delicious. It's hard to resist dunking that bread into the mix — just try to make it whole wheat.

Keeping an eye on mercury

In recent years, there has been a growing concern regarding the methyl mercury content of some fish. Water pollution may increase the level of this metal to toxic amounts in certain areas. The U.S. Food and Drug Administration (FDA) cautions pregnant and nursing women, as well as women of childbearing age, to limit consumption of swordfish, shark, king mackerel, and tile fish to less than 7 ounces per week. These fish are shown to have the greatest mercury levels compared with other fish species. Ahi tuna is generally considered to be safe. However, if you're concerned about the mercury content of fish, visit www.fda.gov to find out more.

AltaMare Fish Soup

Prep time: 30 min • **Cook time:** 6–8 min • **Yield:** 4 servings

Ingredients	Directions
4 cups fish broth	**1** In a medium covered skillet, bring the broth to a boil.
12 little neck clams, cleaned and scrubbed	**2** Add the clams and dashi powder, and cook on medium until the clams open.
1 teaspoon dry dashi powder (Japanese soup stock powder)	**3** Add the rest of the ingredients, boil for 2 more minutes, and serve in soup bowls.
4 baby bok choy, cut lengthwise	
8 ounces rock shrimp, cleaned and deveined	
4 ounces calamari, cleaned and cut in rings	
1 ounce Enoki mushrooms	
1 teaspoon chopped fresh ginger	
1 teaspoon chopped fresh scallion	

Per serving: Kcalories 182 (From Fat 15); Fat 1.5g (Saturated 0g); Cholesterol 2mg; Sodium 868mg; Carbohydrate 5.5g (Dietary Fiber 1.5g); Protein 31g.

Horseradish-Crusted Cod with Lentils

Prep time: 20 min • **Cook time:** 30 min • **Yield:** 4 servings

Ingredients	Directions
1 pound Puy lentils (or substitute the lentils of your choice) 2 sprigs fresh parsley 4 tablespoons crème fraîche (or substitute 3 tablespoons heavy cream and 1 tablespoon sour cream) ¼ cup chopped fresh parsley Salt and pepper 4 teaspoons horseradish sauce 4 cod fillets, 6 ounces each 4 tablespoons panko bread crumbs (substitute crushed cornflakes if you can't find these Japanese bread crumbs in the Asian section of your market) 1 teaspoon olive oil	*1* Preheat the oven to 375 degrees. Place the lentils in a large saucepan with enough cold water to cover them, plus an extra couple of inches. Add the whole sprigs of the parsley and bring to a boil. Simmer for 25 minutes, or until tender. Discard the parsley sprigs. Drain the lentils and toss with the crème fraîche and chopped parsley. Season to taste. Set aside and keep warm. *2* Spread the horseradish sauce over each fish fillet and then press in the bread crumbs to coat. Grease a nonstick baking sheet with the olive oil. Place the fish fillets on the baking sheet and bake for 14 to 17 minutes, until the fish is just cooked and the bread crumbs are golden. *3* Place one-fourth of the lentils on each of four plates. Top each with one piece of baked fish.

Per serving: Kcalories 590 (From Fat 77); Fat 9g (Saturated 4g); Cholesterol 81mg; Sodium 281mg; Carbohydrate 73g (Dietary Fiber 26g); Protein 58g.

Poached King Salmon with Steamed Asparagus and Tapenade Salsa

Prep time: 45 min • **Cook time:** 15 min • **Yield:** 4 servings

Ingredients	Directions
Fish Stock (see the following recipe)	**1** Prepare the fish stock.
½ pound green asparagus	**2** While the stock is cooking, prepare the asparagus. Add the asparagus to lightly salted, boiling water and cook until tender. Immediately remove the asparagus from the boiling water and shock it in a cold-water bath. (Check out Chapter 11 for tips on blanching and shocking vegetables.)
½ pound white asparagus (if not available, use an additional ½ pound green asparagus)	
4 salmon fillets, 6 ounces each	**3** Bring prepared fish stock to a gentle simmer over medium heat. Add the salmon fillets to the simmering fish stock and cook for 5 minutes. Remove from broth and keep warm.
Tapenade Salsa (see the accompanying recipe)	
	4 Prepare the tapenade salsa (see the accompanying recipe).
	5 Just before serving, reheat the asparagus in the simmering fish stock, approximately 5 minutes.
	6 Serve each salmon fillet with the asparagus tips and top with the Tapenade Salsa.

Fish Stock

1 pound fish bones	*1*	In a large sauté pan, add the fish bones to 1 cup of cold water and bring to a simmer.
2 cups water, divided		
1 small onion, diced	*2*	Add the onion, leeks, clove, and white wine and return to a simmer; then add the remaining 1 cup water and the lemon juice. Continue to cook the bones for an additional 30 minutes.
½ pound leeks, sliced and well rinsed		
1 pinch ground cloves		
¼ cup dry white wine	*3*	Strain the broth through a fine mesh strainer. Reserve the broth; discard the bones and other solids.
Juice of 1 lemon		

Tip: You can purchase fish bones at fish markets or at specialty food stores that sell fresh fish. Alternatively, you can find a fish stock base, like Redi-Base, on the web at `www.redibase.com/about.htm#redibase`. It's a concentrate version of stock.

Tapenade Salsa

2 ounces anchovies	*1*	In a food processor, combine the anchovies, olives, and garlic until the mixture becomes a paste, about 45 seconds.
1 cup pitted black olives		
2 cloves garlic		
1 cup olive oil	*2*	In a separate bowl, combine the olive oil and vinegar.
2 tablespoons balsamic vinegar	*3*	Combine the two mixtures and stir.

Per serving: Kcalories 838 (From Fat 639); Fat 71g (Saturated 10g); Cholesterol 109mg; Sodium 1,226mg; Carbohydrate 7g (Dietary Fiber 1g); Protein 43g.

Tip: If you don't have the time or energy to prepare your own fish stock, you can find the prepared version at many grocery stores and specialty food stores. Just remember, homemade always tastes better and is better for you, too!

Tilapia Franchaise

Prep time: 10 min • **Cook time:** 15 min • **Yield:** 2 servings

Ingredients	*Directions*
Nonstick cooking spray	*1* Coat a medium skillet with the cooking spray and place over medium heat.
2 pieces (6 ounces each) tilapia (or other flat white fish)	
1 egg	*2* Rinse and dry the tilapia. In a small bowl, lightly beat the egg. Place the flour in a flat plate. Lightly coat both sides of the fish with the flour, coat the fish with the egg, and place directly in the hot skillet.
½ cup whole-wheat flour	
¼ cup white cooking wine	
1 tablespoon lemon juice	*3* When the fish is golden brown on the first side (approximately 4 minutes), flip it over to brown the other side.
½ cup low-salt chicken broth	
	4 When the fish is golden brown (roughly after 2 to 3 minutes), reduce the heat to low. Add the wine and let it reduce to half the amount. Add the lemon juice and broth and let the liquid reduce as it cooks the fish.
	5 When the liquid has reduced to approximately one quarter and appears to have slightly thickened, remove from the heat and serve.

Per serving: Kcalories 291(From Fat 45); Fat 5g (Saturated 2g); Cholesterol 190mg; Sodium 156mg; Carbohydrate 23g (Dietary Fiber 4g); Protein 40g.

Tip: Serve with fresh vegetables, salad, whole-wheat couscous, or brown rice for some extra fiber.

Salmon Steaks Vinaigrette

Prep time: 20 min • **Cook time:** 10 min • **Yield:** 4 servings

Ingredients	Directions
4 salmon steaks, about 1½ inches thick	*1* Preheat the oven on broil.
Salt and pepper to taste	*2* Sprinkle the salmon with the salt and pepper.
2 tablespoons olive oil	
3 tablespoons red wine vinegar	*3* In a large bowl, combine the remaining ingredients to make a vinaigrette.
1 teaspoon Italian herbs	*4* Marinate the salmon in the vinaigrette for 20 minutes.
½ teaspoon paprika	
1 teaspoon grated onion	*5* Transfer the salmon to a foil-lined pan.
2 tablespoons lemon juice	*6* Broil about 6 inches from a preheated broiler 5 to 7 minutes, until the fish flakes.
	7 Turn the salmon and broil another 5 to 7 minutes, to brown both sides.

Per serving: Kcalories 255 (From Fat 153); Fat 17g (Saturated 3g); Cholesterol 109mg; Sodium 70mg; Carbohydrate 53g (Dietary Fiber 0g); Protein 30g.

Pan-Roasted Cod with Shrimp and Mirliton Squash

Prep time: 1 hr • **Cook time:** 40 min • **Yield:** 4 servings

Ingredients	*Directions*
Fumet:	*1* Preheat the oven to 350 degrees. Place the shrimp shells, shallot, bay leaf, thyme, Chardonnay, and enough water to cover the ingredients in a small sauce-pot. Slowly bring to a boil and simmer for 15 to 20 minutes to extract some flavor from the shells. After the flavor has been extracted, strain the liquid. Discard the shells and other solids and reserve the liquid.
Shrimp shells, from twenty 26/30 shrimp (from shrimp in ragoût or purchased at a local fish market; see the note at the end of the recipe)	
1 shallot, chopped	
1 bay leaf	*2* Make the ragoût: In a medium saucepan, place the shrimp, squash, tomato, fumet, butter, lemon juice, salt, and parsley. Simmer until the shrimp is done, approximately 5 to 7 minutes, and hold until ready to serve. Adjust seasoning as needed.
1 thyme sprig	
½ cup Chardonnay	
Ragoût:	
20 white shrimp, 26/30s, peeled and deveined	*3* Lightly season the cod fillets with salt and pepper to taste and dust one side with flour.
2 cups ¼-inch cubes of peeled chayote squash (also called mirliton), blanched (see Chapter 11 for blanching instructions)	
1 cup peeled, cubed tomato	
½ cup Shrimp Fumet	

2 tablespoons butter

2 teaspoons fresh lemon juice

1 teaspoon kosher salt

2 tablespoons parsley (whole leaves)

Cod:

4 cod fillets (6 ounces each)

Salt and pepper

2 teaspoons flour

2 tablespoons olive oil

4 Heat the olive oil in a sauté pan and place the cod fillets flour side down in the oil. Sauté to a golden brown, approximately 4 minutes, and then turn and transfer to the oven for 4 to 6 minutes.

5 When the cod is finished baking in the oven, place each fillet in a bowl and pour the ragoût on top.

Per serving: Kcalories 292 (From Fat 126); Fat 14g (Saturated 5g); Cholesterol 134mg; Sodium 776mg; Carbohydrate 7g (Dietary Fiber 2g); Protein 34g.

Note: Shrimp fall into various size categories, and 26/30 means you get 26 to 30 shrimp in each pound. For more information, see Chapter 7.

Note: A *fumet* (pronounced foo-MAY) is a heavily concentrated stock. In the case of this recipe, it's a stock made from shrimp shells. You can make a fumet by boiling fish heads, bones, shellfish shells, or whole fish with wine, aromatic herbs, and vegetables and then reducing it to concentrate the flavor. Use a fumet to season sauces and soups or to braise or poach fish or vegetables. Its subtle flavor imparts the delicate essence of seafood with a slight acidity (thanks to the wine), but it doesn't overpower the main event. If you'd rather not make your own fumet, look for fish stock or fish stock glace or base (an even more concentrated product that must be reconstituted with water before using) at your local fish or gourmet market.

Tip: Mirliton squash, also known as chayote squash, is similar to other squash varieties. Look for a small, avocado-sized squash with a firm pale green skin. It has a white mild-flavored flesh that takes on the subtle flavors of the shrimp fumet very well. Its peak season runs from December to March, so if you can't find it, zucchini works well too.

Halibut in Parchment

Prep time: 15 min • **Cook time:** 25 min • **Yield:** 2 servings

Ingredients	Directions
2 teaspoons chopped cilantro 1 shallot, diced 1 large zucchini, sliced 1 large yellow squash, sliced 1 large tomato, quartered Salt and pepper to taste 2 halibut filets 1 small lemon	**1** Preheat the oven to 375 degrees. **2** In a medium bowl, combine the cilantro, shallot, zucchini, squash, tomato, pinch of salt, and pepper. **3** Put each halibut filet on a 12-inch square of parchment paper, dust with salt and pepper, and top with the vegetable mixture. Slice the lemon and fan it on top of the vegetables. **4** Fold the halibut in the parchment paper and roll the edges to close. Place on a cookie sheet and cook for 20 to 25 minutes.

Per serving: Kcalories 196 (From Fat 27); Fat 3g (Saturated .5g); Cholesterol 95mg; Sodium 92mg; Carbohydrate 15g (Dietary Fiber 4g); Protein 28g.

Tip: Cooking in parchment is probably the easiest way to cook fish while preserving its taste. The fish will take on the flavors of whatever you put in the parchment with it, so you can vary this recipe in numerous ways according to your taste. Halibut by itself tends to be somewhat bland, so feel free to be creative. Additional benefits of cooking in parchment include no sticking of the fish to a grill, no loss of other ingredients through the grill, and wonderful odors when you open the parchment.

Swordfish with Lemon Salsa

Prep time: 20 min, plus marinade time • **Cook time:** 10 min • **Yield:** 6 servings

Ingredients	Directions
2 tablespoons finely diced shallot	*1* Preheat the oven to 400 degrees.
1 tablespoon champagne vinegar	*2* In a large bowl, combine all ingredients except the fish and lemon.
½ cup juice from Meyer lemons	*3* Marinate the swordfish steaks for at least 2 hours.
1½ cups Castelvetrano olives, medium dice	*4* Remove the fish from the marinade. Pat dry. Place on a heavy metal baking pan and transfer to the oven. Cook for 10 minutes.
2 tablespoons chopped parsley	
⅓ cup extra-virgin olive oil	
1 teaspoon honey	*5* Garnish the swordfish with Meyer lemon sections.
Salt and pepper to taste	
Six 4-ounce swordfish steaks	
Meyer lemon, for garnish	

Per serving: Kcalories 196 (From Fat 27); Fat 3g (Saturated .5g); Cholesterol 95mg; Sodium 92mg; Carbohydrate 15g (Dietary Fiber 4g); Protein 28g.

Note: Swordfish is delicious, but there is some concern about eating too much of it because it contains mercury. Recent studies don't seem to confirm a harmful effect of mercury on the heart, but it may affect a baby's developing brain, so it isn't advised for a woman who is pregnant or may become pregnant. The rest of us can enjoy swordfish as one of a variety of different fishes. The health benefits of eating fish far outweigh the danger.

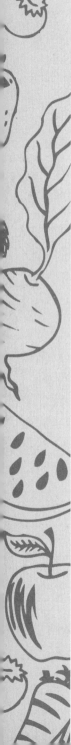

Grouper Acquapazza

Prep time: 15 min • **Cook time:** 15 min • **Yield:** 2 servings

Ingredients	*Directions*
1 tablespoon olive oil	*1* In a nonstick 12-inch pan, add the olive oil and heat until hot.
Two 8-ounce filets of grouper, skin on	
2 garlic cloves, chopped	*2* Place the fish filet in the pan and sear on each side for approximately 2 minutes.
1 tablespoon capers	
2 tablespoons black olives (preferably Taggiasca)	*3* Add the garlic, capers, and olives to the pan, and stir for 1 minute.
2 fresh plum tomatoes, seeded and chopped	
One 16-ounce can San Marzano peeled tomatoes, drained and chopped	*4* Add both tomatoes and the fish broth to the pan. Let cook for another 5 to 6 minutes.
10 ounces fish broth (or substitute ½ cup clam juice and 6 ounces water)	*5* Transfer the filets to a hot plate.
	6 Continue to cook the sauce for 2 to 3 more minutes or until thickened.
1 bunch fresh basil, chopped	
Salt and pepper to taste	*7* Stir in the basil and pour over the fish.

Per serving: Kcalories 230 (From Fat 81); Fat 9g (Saturated 2g); Cholesterol 95mg; Sodium 913mg; Carbohydrate 15g (Dietary Fiber 4g); Protein 27g.

B.B.Q. Cedar-Planked Salmon

Prep time: 30 min, plus plank soaking time of 2 hr • **Cook time:** 20 min • **Yield:** 6 servings

Ingredients	Directions
½ **tablespoon salt**	*1* Soak a cedar plank in water for at least 2 hours. The plank should measure 1 to 2 inches larger than salmon fillet all the way around.
½ **cup brown sugar**	
Zest from 1 orange	*2* Preheat the oven to 450 degrees.
1 salmon fillet (2 pounds), pin bone removed (ask the person at the seafood counter to do this for you)	*3* Mix up the dry marinade. In a small bowl mix the salt, brown sugar, and orange zest and spread it generously on both sides of the salmon fillet. (You can marinate the fish 1 to 2 hours in advance, if you prefer. Refrigerate the fish while it's marinating if you marinate it in advance.)
5 tablespoons olive oil, divided	
6 garlic cloves, finely chopped	
½ **cup chiffonade basil (roll the basil together tightly and then thinly slice width-wise to form long, stringy strips)**	*4* Brush one side of the cedar plank with 3 tablespoons of the olive oil and place it in the oven for 15 to 20 minutes.
1 large onion, peeled and thinly sliced	*5* Spread the garlic on the olive-oil-coated side of the plank and then place the salmon fillet on top. Sprinkle the salmon fillet with the basil. Cover the fish generously with the sliced onions and then drizzle it with the remaining 2 tablespoons olive oil.
	6 Place the planked fish in the preheated oven. Cook the salmon for approximately 10 to 15 minutes, or until the fish is medium-rare and a probe thermometer reads 120 degrees. The cooking time will vary with the thickness of your fish. Allow approximately 10 minutes per inch of thickness.

Per serving: Kcalories 373 (From Fat 153); Fat 17g (Saturated 2g); Cholesterol 86mg; Sodium 700mg; Carbohydrate 21g (Dietary Fiber 1g); Protein 33g.

Tip: You can find cedar planks at a lumber store — specifically look for untreated cedar shingles — or in kitchen supply stores or gourmet shops that sell lots of knickknacks.

Tip: If you prefer to cook the salmon on a grill, follow these instructions: Preheat the grill to medium-high heat. Place the oiled plank directly on the grill. Let the plank smoke a bit before adding the fish. If the plank catches on fire, spritz it with water. Close the grill and cook the salmon for approximately 10 to 15 minutes, or until the fish is medium-rare and a probe thermometer reads 120 degrees. The cooking time will vary with the thickness of your fish. Allow approximately 10 minutes per inch of thickness.

Grilled Ahi Tuna with Asian Slaw

Prep time: 30 min plus 2 hr for marinating • **Cook time:** 6–10 min • **Yield:** 4 servings

Ingredients	Directions
4 ahi tuna steaks, about 2 pounds (be sure they're sushi grade)	**1** Make the marinade by combining the soy sauce, mirin, sesame oil, vinegar, gingerroot, green onions, and garlic in a resealable plastic bag. Place the ahi steaks in the bag. Gently coat the steaks in the marinade. Place in the refrigerator for 2 hours, turning occasionally.
Marinade:	
¼ cup light soy sauce	
¼ cup mirin (sweet rice wine)	**2** About a half hour before the ahi has finished marinating, prepare the slaw: First mix the dressing ingredients (vinegar, Splenda, honey, soy sauce, cilantro, gingerroot, and sesame seeds) in a large bowl. In another large bowl, mix the slaw ingredients (cabbage, carrots, onion, red and yellow bell peppers, and radish). Toss the cabbage mixture with most of the dressing. Reserve a small amount of dressing for later.
1 tablespoon toasted sesame oil	
2 tablespoons rice wine vinegar	
2 tablespoons minced fresh gingerroot	
2½ tablespoons minced green onions	**3** Let stand for 20 minutes at room temperature. If you'd prefer to refrigerate the slaw, extend standing time to 1 hour (and start preparing it about 40 minutes after you start marinating the tuna). Preheat the grill.
3 tablespoons minced garlic	
Dressing:	
⅔ cup rice wine vinegar	**4** Grill the ahi tuna 2 to 3 minutes per side. (Broil about 5 inches from the heating element, if you prefer.) The outside should be gray brown; however, the inside will remain red. Be sure not to overcook the steaks, as they will quickly dry out and lose flavor.
½ tablespoon Splenda (or to taste)	
1 teaspoon honey	
1 teaspoon light soy sauce	
3 tablespoons chopped cilantro	
1 teaspoon finely grated gingerroot	
1 tablespoon toasted sesame seeds	

Slaw:

1 small head Napa cabbage, shredded

½ cup shredded carrot

¼ cup chopped green onion

¼ cup julienned red bell pepper

¼ cup julienned yellow bell pepper

½ cup julienned daikon radish

5 Slice the tuna thinly and serve with the slaw. Drizzle the reserved dressing on top.

Per serving of ahi tuna: Kcalories 258 (From Fat 27); Fat 3g (Saturated 1g); Cholesterol 99mg; Sodium 232mg; Carbohydrate 2g (Dietary Fiber 0g); Protein 51g.

Per serving of slaw and dressing: Kcalories 57 (from Fat 12); Fat 1g (Saturated 0 g); Cholesterol 0 mg; Sodium 73mg; Carbohydrate 10g (Dietary Fiber 3g); Protein 3g.

Note: Fresh tuna is best when prepared very rare in the middle — nearly raw. For this reason, be sure to purchase sushi-grade tuna at the fish market. It's safer, less likely to be contaminated, and therefore less likely to cause food-borne illness. Pregnant and nursing women should always avoid all raw fish, including rare tuna. Otherwise, be sure to meet the American Heart Association's recommendation to consume 2 servings of fish per week.

Surveying Superior Shellfish

The term *shellfish* includes seafood such as shrimp, lobster, oysters, clams, mussels, and scallops, which all have a shell instead of fins and gills. It also includes some seafood that have a not-so-obvious shell, like octopus and squid.

Shellfish are sold by their size and weight. For tips on how to pick the right shellfish for your recipe, check out Chapter 7.

The texture of these tasty tidbits ranges from exceptionally tender, in the case of lobster and some shrimp, to a bit chewy, in the case of octopus. It's probably not a surprise that the tenderness of these delicate creatures depends, in part, on how well you cook them.

Avoid overcooking shellfish. Doing so causes the texture to become rubbery and unpleasant.

Rock Shrimp Ceviche

Prep time: 10 min • **Marinating time:** 1 hr • **Yield:** 4 servings

Ingredients	Directions
1 pound rock shrimp, roughly chopped	Place the rock shrimp in a bowl and mix together with the mango, shallot, cilantro, lime juice, and chili flakes. Season with salt and pepper to taste and place in the refrigerator for 1 hour. The ceviche looks particularly attractive served in a martini glass.
1 mango, small dice	
1 shallot, finely chopped	
½ cup chopped fresh cilantro	
½ cup fresh lime juice (about 4 limes)	
1 pinch chili flakes	
Salt and pepper	

Per serving: Kcalories 131 (From Fat 10); Fat 1g (Saturated 0g); Cholesterol 168mg; Sodium 340mg; Carbohydrate 13g (Dietary Fiber 1g); Protein 19g.

Note: Use only very fresh (or freshly frozen and then very recently thawed) seafood in ceviche because it never reaches temperatures high enough to kill strong bacteria.

Fettuccini Shrimp

Prep time: 15 min • **Cook time:** 15–20 min • **Yield:** 2 servings

Ingredients	*Directions*
4 ounces fettuccini	*1* In a large pot, boil the pasta in salted water until al dente.
1 tablespoon olive oil	
2 garlic cloves, sliced	*2* Meanwhile, in a large pan, heat the oil and sauté the garlic and asparagus for 3 minutes.
2 ounces asparagus, chopped	
2 ounces snow peas	*3* Add the shrimp and snow peas to the pan and cook for 30 seconds to a minute.
6 ounces rock shrimp	
Salt and pepper to taste	*4* Toss in the fettuccini, season with salt and pepper, and serve.

Per serving: Kcalories 475 (From Fat 63); Fat 9g (Saturated 1g); Cholesterol 165mg; Sodium 118mg; Carbohydrate 73g (Dietary Fiber 7g); Protein 25g.

Tip: Don't overcook the shrimp — it can quickly lose its flavor with too much cooking. You know it's cooked sufficiently when it curls and develops a little color.

Seared Diver Scallops with Bacon and Shallot Reduction

Prep time: 30 min • **Cook time:** 30 min • **Yield:** 2 servings

Ingredients	Directions
4 slices slab bacon, cut into ½-inch strips 1 shallot, peeled and thinly sliced ½ cup low-sodium chicken stock 2 tablespoons butter 1 tablespoon chopped fresh chives Salt and pepper 6 U10 diver scallops (you can substitute 1 pound of sea scallops) 2 tablespoons olive oil 12 asparagus stalks (approximately ¼ pound), cleaned, trimmed, and blanched (see Chapter 11 for blanching instructions) ¼ cup Balsamic Syrup (see the accompanying recipe)	**1** Add the bacon to a small sauté pan and cook for 2 minutes. Add the shallots and continue cooking for an additional 3 minutes. Add the chicken stock and butter and bring to a simmer until the stock has reduced by half and the onions are tender, approximately 20 minutes. Add the chives and season to taste with salt and pepper. Set aside. **2** Preheat a medium sauté pan over high heat. Season the scallops evenly on both sides with salt and pepper. Add the oil to the hot pan and sauté the scallops approximately 2 minutes per side. Remove the scallops from the pan and place 3 scallops in the center of each plate. Reheat the asparagus in the skillet you used to cook the scallops. Put the bacon and shallot reduction (from Step 1) around the scallops. Arrange the asparagus around the scallops. Drizzle the Balsamic Syrup over the scallops and asparagus.

Balsamic Syrup

1 cup balsamic vinegar 1½ teaspoons Splenda	Combine the balsamic vinegar and Splenda in a medium saucepan. Cook over medium-high heat until the sauce thickens and reduces to ¼ cup, approximately 30 minutes.

Per serving of scallops: Kcalories 652 (From Fat 306); Fat 34g (Saturated 11g); Cholesterol 154mg; Sodium 1,090mg; Carbohydrate 29g (Dietary Fiber 2g); Protein 52g.

Per serving of Balsamic Syrup (2 tablespoons): Kcalories 80 (From Fat 2); Fat 0g (Saturated 0g); Cholesterol 0mg; Sodium 31mg; Carbohydrate 19g (Dietary Fiber 0g); Protein 0g.

Tip: Serve this dish atop a bed of whole-wheat couscous to complete the meal.

Fresh Jumbo Lump Crabmeat with Wild Rice Sautéed in Sherry

Prep time: 1 hr 15 min • **Cook time:** 1 hr 10 min • **Yield:** 4 servings

Ingredients	Directions
6 tablespoons butter	**1** Place two skillets on a stove over medium heat.
4 tablespoons extra-virgin olive oil	**2** Add 3 tablespoons of butter to each skillet, let it melt, and add 2 tablespoons of olive oil to each skillet. One skillet will be used for preparing the wild rice and the other will be used for the crabmeat.
1 small shallot, thinly sliced	
Salt and pepper to taste	
1 cup cooked wild rice	**3** In the first skillet, add the shallots and a pinch of salt and pepper. Sauté for 2 to 3 minutes. Add the cooked wild rice and stir.
16 ounces fresh jumbo crabmeat	
8 ounces sherry drinking wine, divided equally	**4** In the second skillet, add the crabmeat.
	5 To each skillet, add 4 ounces of sherry wine and cook until the alcohol reduces in volume by half.
	6 Stir both skillets in order for everything to mix well.
	7 Place the wild rice on one side of a plate and the crabmeat on the other side. Drizzle the sherry wine sauce from the crabmeat skillet over the crabmeat.

Per serving: Kcalories 347 (From Fat 135); Fat 15g (Saturated 2g); Cholesterol 48mg; Sodium 955mg; Carbohydrate 16g (Dietary Fiber 0g); Protein 23g.

Chawan Mushi Egg Custard and Clams

Prep time: 20 min • **Cook time:** 35 min • **Yield:** 6 servings

Ingredients	Directions
12 Manila clams	*1* Preheat the oven to 300 degrees.
2 eggs	
6 morel mushrooms, sliced	*2* In a medium saucepan, steam the clams in 1 cup water, covered, for 4 to 5 minutes, until they open.
½ cup peas, sliced	
¼ cup pine nuts	*3* Remove the clams from the saucepan and allow them to cool. Chop them up.
2 scallions, diced	
1 cup dashi broth (prepared using dashi powder available online or at specialty markets)	*4* Strain and cool the liquid, saving 1 cup. Whisk the liquid into the eggs, and season with the dashi broth.
	5 Distribute the mushrooms, peas, pine nuts, scallions, and clams between 6 ramekins. Ladle 2½ ounces of the egg mixture into each.
	6 Place the cups in a roasting pan, and add boiling water halfway up the sides.
	7 Bake for 30 to 40 minutes, until set.

Per serving: Kcalories 119 (From Fat 72); Fat 8g (Saturated 1.5g); Cholesterol 6mg; Sodium 97mg; Carbohydrate 4g (Dietary Fiber 1g); Protein 9g.

Chapter 13

Poultry: Moist and Delicious

When you first received your diagnosis of diabetes, you may have assumed that your culinary life would include nothing more than broiled chicken breasts and steamed vegetables. Hopefully, if you've read any of this book at this point, you realize this assumption couldn't be farther from reality.

In this chapter, we show you how to safely use poultry in your diet. We give you tips to keep the most popular piece of chicken — the breast — tasty, moist, and downright exciting. And finally, we give you some great ways to include turkey in your regimen.

Including Poultry in Your Diet

Nutritionists define a portion as 3.5 ounces. What this serving size looks like on your dinner plate, with chicken for instance, is typically either a half chicken breast or a chicken drumstick and thigh. To reduce the fat content, eat the meat but don't eat the skin.

Maintaining good sanitary practices in your kitchen is important when you're working with poultry, no matter how much poultry you're cooking. Keep the following hints in mind to minimize bacterial contamination from poultry:

✔ Rinse any poultry pieces and pat them dry before using them. This step helps remove bacteria that are often present in poultry.

✔ Don't place raw poultry near, over, or in any foods that won't be cooked before they're eaten. Proper cooking kills most bacteria found in poultry, but never let the liquid in raw poultry drip onto salads, sauces, condiments, and the like.

✔ Keep a separate color cutting board only used for raw poultry. You can significantly reduce the chances that you cut lettuce on the same board you sliced chicken on if they're different colors.

✔ Clean your knife after cutting raw poultry. Wash it thoroughly in hot, soapy water.

✔ Thoroughly sanitize any surfaces that come into contact with any raw poultry or its juices. Use an antibacterial cleaner that's specifically made for this purpose.

✔ Always cook poultry to the appropriate food-safe temperature, as listed in Table 13-1.

Table 13-1	Safe Cooking Temperatures for Poultry
Product	*Temperature*
Ground turkey, chicken	165
Poultry breasts	170
Chicken, whole	180
Duck and goose	180
Poultry thighs, wings	180
Turkey, whole	180

Making the Best of Chicken Breasts

The breast is the leanest of all the chicken's parts, with the lowest total and saturated fat content, thus making it the healthiest choice for your heart.

Chicken Breasts with Lemon and Garlic

Prep time: 20 min • **Cook time:** 25 min • **Yield:** 6 servings

Ingredients	*Directions*
6 chicken breasts, 6 ounces each, bone in, with skin **Salt** **2 tablespoons extra-virgin olive oil, divided** **30 garlic cloves** **4 tablespoons butter** **Juice of 2 lemons, divided** **1 cup dry white wine** **3 cups chicken stock or water** **A few thyme sprigs** **Zest of 1 lemon, divided**	*1* A few hours before cooking, season the chicken breasts with salt. Refrigerate the chicken and bring to room temperature when ready to use.
	2 In a small sauté pan, heat 1 tablespoon of the olive oil and add the garlic. Cook it over medium-low heat, allowing it to brown but not burn. Shake the pan occasionally or stir the garlic with a spoon to keep it from burning. Add a little water if the garlic starts to brown too much. Cook the garlic until it is soft, about 15 to 20 minutes.
	3 Once the garlic is soft, in a large Dutch oven over medium heat, heat the remaining olive oil and 2 tablespoons of butter and slowly brown the chicken, skin side down, until the skin is golden and crisp. Turn the breasts over and reduce the heat to medium-low.
	4 Once you flip the breasts, add the garlic and olive oil sauce to the chicken pan. Add half the lemon juice, the white wine, the chicken stock, the thyme, and half the lemon zest. Bring the sauce to a simmer and cover. Continue cooking for approximately 5 to 7 minutes, or until the breasts are cooked through and tender, but not dried out. Check the chicken and sauce occasionally, stirring as needed. If the pan begins to dry, add a little water to maintain about a half-inch of liquid in the pan.
	5 When the chicken is cooked and its juices run clear, remove it from the pan to a warm serving platter. Keep warm. Increase the heat in the skillet until the sauce begins to boil, and then shut off the heat and add the remaining 2 tablespoons butter. Adjust the seasonings with salt, pepper, and the remaining lemon juice, if desired. Pour the sauce over the chicken.
	6 Garnish with the remaining lemon zest. Remove the chicken skin before eating.

Per serving: *Kcalories 288 (From Fat 153); Fat 17g (Saturated 7g); Cholesterol 91mg; Sodium 660mg; Carbohydrate 7g (Dietary Fiber 1g); Protein 26g.*

Grilled Summer Chicken Tartare

Prep time: 25 min • **Cook time:** 10 min • **Yield:** 8 servings

Ingredients	Directions
2 pounds grilled skinless chicken breast, seasoned with salt and pepper and diced into small cubes	*1* In a large bowl, combine all ingredients and adjust with salt, pepper, and additional lime juice if necessary.
1 white onion, diced small	*2* Serve with a small toasted pita cut into triangles for an additional 150 calories and 2 grams of fat.
2 bunches cilantro, chopped	
¼ cup crema Mexicana	
½ cup fresh squeezed lime juice	
2 tablespoons extra-virgin olive oil	
2 cups cherry tomatoes, quartered	
1 avocado, cut into small cubes	

Per serving: Kcalories 305 (From Fat 126); Fat 14g (Saturated 3g); Cholesterol 105mg; Sodium 121mg; Carbohydrate 7g (Dietary Fiber 3g); Protein 37g.

Note: Crema Mexicana, a topping used in a wide variety of Mexican dishes, is cultured sour cream cheese prepared with pasteurized milk. It has a creamier texture than sour cream. It's like the Mexican version of French crème fraîche but smoother. You can use it in other recipes in place of sour cream — for example, on potatoes, in soups, and on tacos.

West African Braised Chicken

Prep time: 35 min • **Cook time:** 2 hr 20 min • **Yield:** 6 servings

Ingredients	*Directions*
2 pounds bone-in chicken thighs, skin removed	*1* Season the chicken with kosher salt and pepper.
Kosher salt to taste	
Pepper to taste	*2* In a large stainless-steel stock pot, brown the chicken thighs in olive oil. Remove from pot and set aside.
1 tablespoon olive oil	
2 medium yellow onions, diced small	*3* In the same pot (do not clean), sauté the onions, garlic, ginger, turmeric, fennel and chile de árbol until translucent. Add the tomato puree and peanut butter and cook until warm.
6 cloves whole garlic	
½ cup ginger brunoise (very finely diced ginger)	
6 chile de árbol, chopped and soaked in hot water for 30 minutes	*4* Stir in the toasted coriander, cumin, cinnamon, and pepper.
4 tablespoons tomato puree	*5* Add vegetable stock and diced tomatoes and continue to cook for about 5 minutes.
½ cup all-natural peanut butter	
2 teaspoons toasted coriander	*6* Add the chicken back in and cook for 2 hours at low to medium heat.
1 teaspoon cumin	
½ teaspoon ground cinnamon	*7* When the chicken is cooked and starting to pull away, add the charred Japanese eggplant and charred okra.
1 teaspoon pepper	
2 cups vegetable stock	*8* Serve with brown rice, whole-wheat couscous, or your favorite grain.
2 cups diced tomatoes	
1½ pounds Japanese eggplant, seasoned and charred in a cast-iron pan and diced small	
8 ounces charred fresh okra, seasoned with salt and pepper and charred in a cast-iron pan and diced small	
2 teaspoons turmeric	
1 teaspoon toasted fennel	

Per serving: *Kcalories 385 (From Fat 144); Fat 18g (Saturated 4g); Cholesterol 180mg; Sodium 335mg; Carbohydrate 20g (Dietary Fiber 6g); Protein 33g.*

Chicken Scampi

Prep time: 6–7 hr (mostly marinating time) • **Cook time:** 20–30 min • **Yield:** 4 servings

Ingredients	Directions
¼ teaspoon pepper	*1* Combine the pepper, half the garlic, the salt, oregano, parsley, lemon juice, and half of the wine in a resealable plastic bag. Add the chicken. Mix gently to coat the chicken with the marinade. Marinate in the refrigerator for several hours (overnight is best).
2 cloves garlic, minced, divided	
¼ teaspoon salt	
2 tablespoons roughly chopped fresh oregano	*2* When ready to cook the chicken, preheat the broiler, on low if your range has this setting. Remove the chicken from the marinade (save the remaining marinade) and place in a shallow pan. Broil 8 inches from the heat, turning once, until the chicken is no longer pink inside (about 15 minutes).
¼ cup roughly chopped fresh parsley	
3 tablespoons lemon juice	
¼ cup white wine, divided	
5 skinless, boneless chicken breast halves, 4 ounces each, cut into 1-inch strips	*3* While the chicken is broiling, heat the olive oil in a sauté pan. Sauté the remaining garlic, until fragrant, but not browned. Add the remaining white wine to the sauté pan and scrape to remove any bits on the pan. Add the remaining marinade and chicken stock. Bring to a boil. Reduce the sauce by half. Stir in the butter and tomatoes. Season with salt and pepper, as needed. Pour the sauce over the chicken. Top with the Parmesan cheese.
1 tablespoon olive oil	
¼ cup chicken stock	
1 tablespoon butter	
½ cup Roma tomatoes, diced	
Salt and pepper to taste	
3 tablespoons grated Parmesan cheese	

Per serving: Kcalories 241 (From Fat 100); Fat 11g (Saturated 4g); Cholesterol 89mg; Sodium 496mg; Carbohydrate 3g (Dietary Fiber 1g); Protein 31g.

Paillard of Chicken Breast with Fennel and Parmigiano

Prep time: 30 min • **Cook time:** 30 min • **Yield:** 4 servings

Ingredients	Directions
1 bunch fresh chives **5 tablespoons extra-virgin olive oil, divided** **Pinch of salt**	*1* Chop the chives. In a blender, blend the chives with 3 tablespoons of olive oil. Add the pinch of salt.
1 bulb fennel	*2* Slice the fennel into paper-thin slices.
4 cups baby arugula **4 ounces Parmigiano, sliced paper thin**	*3* Arrange four dinner plates with baby arugula on one side and fennel slices layered with Parmigiano slices over arugula. Halve the cherry tomatoes and place on either side of the salad.
1¼ pounds cherry tomatoes **Salt and pepper**	*4* Lightly sprinkle salt and pepper on both sides of the chicken breasts.
4 full boneless skinless chicken breasts, 6 ounces each, pounded flat (see the Tip) **3 ounces sun-dried tomatoes in olive oil, pureed** **2 lemons, halved**	*5* Warm the remaining 2 tablespoons of olive oil in a large saucepan. When the pan is very hot, place the 4 chicken breasts in the pan. Cook the breasts until they've acquired a golden color. Flip the breasts over and do the same to the other side. The breasts shouldn't cook more than 2 to 3 minutes on each side. Don't let the breasts become dry.
	6 Place 1 chicken breast paillard on each plate next to the salad. Season with salt and pepper. With a spoon or squirt bottle, dribble the chive sauce and the tomatoes over and around the chicken breast paillards to create a colorful design.
	7 Dress the plate with a drizzle of olive oil and a lemon half.

Per serving (with 2 tablespoons chive and sun-dried tomato vinaigrette): Kcalories 589 (From Fat 300); Fat 33g (Saturated 9g); Cholesterol 116mg; Sodium 904mg; Carbohydrate 24g (Dietary Fiber 7g); Protein 51g.

Tip: A *paillard* (pronounced *pie*-yarhd) is a fancy French word that basically means a cutlet, or a slice of meat that's been pounded to a thin, even thickness (or thinness depending on your viewpoint). To pound meat flat, place it between two pieces of plastic wrap and pound it with a rolling pin or mallet.

Roast Free-Range Chicken Breast Stuffed with Porcini Mushrooms, Caramelized Leeks, and Pancetta

Prep time: 30 min • **Cook time:** 50 min • **Yield:** 4 servings

Ingredients	*Directions*
½ cup dried porcini mushrooms	*1* Place the oven rack in the lower area of the oven. Preheat the oven to 400 degrees. Set aside a large roasting pan.
2 cups warm water, divided	
3 sun-dried tomatoes	*2* Place the porcini mushrooms in 1 cup of warm water. Let rest for 15 minutes. Repeat the process in a separate cup of water with the sun-dried tomatoes. Strain the porcini from the water and reserve the water. Cut the mushrooms into fine juliennes. Strain the sun-dried tomatoes from the water and discard the water. Cut the tomatoes into fine juliennes.
4 ounces lean pancetta (approximately 8 thin slices), diced	
2 tablespoons butter	
1 medium leek, tough greens removed, rinsed well, diced small	
4 chicken breasts, skin on, boned and tenders removed, about 6 ounces each	*3* Sauté the pancetta in a pan until fat is rendered out, but not browned, 3 to 4 minutes.
Salt and pepper	*4* Heat the butter in a small sauté pan over medium heat. When hot, add the leeks and cook until lightly browned, about 4½ minutes. Add the mushrooms, tomatoes, and pancetta to the sauté pan.
1 teaspoon finely chopped fresh thyme	
4 cups watercress, washed	*5* To assemble the chicken breasts, pull the skin back and season both sides with salt and pepper. Sprinkle with thyme on both sides. Spread about ½ cup of the mushroom mixture over each chicken breast. Cover with skin. Place in the reserved roasting pan. Top the chicken breasts with any additional stuffing mixture that is remaining.
1 tablespoon extra-virgin olive oil	
1 tablespoon balsamic vinegar	
2 cups low-sodium chicken stock	*6* Place in the oven and roast until browned, approximately 25 to 30 minutes. Transfer the chicken to a warm platter.

7 Toss the watercress with the olive oil and vinegar.

8 Deglaze the pan. Combine the porcini mushroom water and chicken stock in the pan used for the chicken. Simmer until reduced to ⅓ cup, about 6 to 8 minutes.

9 Serve the chicken breasts over the watercress and pour the sauce on top.

Per serving: Kcalories 527 (From Fat 266); Fat 30g (Saturated 10g); Cholesterol 145mg; Sodium 846mg; Carbohydrate 15g (Dietary Fiber 4g); Protein 50g.

Note: Although you want to keep the skin on while cooking the chicken, be sure to remove it after you sit down to eat. The skin is full of artery-clogging saturated fat.

Making your own marinade

Marinating chicken for hours or even overnight is a great way to maximize flavor and add moisture to chicken breasts. Make up your own marinades based on what you're in the mood for. Here are some ideas to get you started.

✔ Balsamic vinegar, olive oil, and oregano

✔ Light soy sauce, lime juice, minced garlic, and minced ginger

✔ Lowfat salad dressing, like Italian or Greek vinaigrette

Include an acid of some sort in your marinade to help break down some connective tissue in the meat, making it more tender and helping it to absorb the marinade flavor more completely. Good acid choices include citrus juice and vinegar. The marinade in the following recipe features lemon juice.

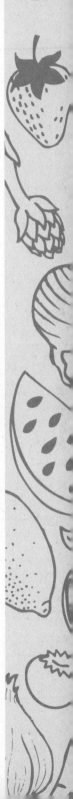

Talking Turkey to Liven Up Your Meals

A standard 3½-ounce serving of white meat turkey, without the skin, has only a gram of saturated fat, which is even less than the same size serving of a chicken breast. Turkey is also a good source of B vitamins and many minerals, including iron, potassium, selenium, and zinc, especially in the dark meat.

If you buy a whole turkey, you tend to get more meat for your money by buying a larger bird. With a small bird, in the 12- to 15-pound range, much of what you get is bones, so you may be disappointed with the meager meat that results from all your hard work. If you have more leftovers than you can (or want to) eat in a couple of days, freeze the extra with a touch of chicken broth to help keep it moist.

"Rotisserie"-Roasted Turkey Breast

Prep time: 20 min • **Cook time:** 2 hr 15 min • **Yield:** Varies based on weight of turkey, 6-ounce serving size

Ingredients	Directions
1 tablespoon olive oil 1 turkey breast, 6 to 7 pounds, with skin 4 tablespoons lemon pepper 1 tablespoon ground sage	*1* Preheat the oven to 400 degrees. Rub the olive oil into the turkey breast. Place the turkey breast in a roasting pan with a rack. (If you don't have a rack, roll up 6 balls of foil and then place under the turkey in the roasting pan to elevate the turkey breast.) To get a rotisserie-like final product, you need to make sure the turkey doesn't sit in any fat as it cooks. Set aside.
	2 In a small bowl, combine the lemon pepper and ground sage. Sprinkle the combined seasonings evenly over oiled turkey breast. Place the roasting pan in the oven. Cook for 45 minutes at 400 degrees. Then reduce the oven temperature to 300 degrees to finish cooking, approximately 1½ hours, depending on the size of your bird. Cook the turkey until it reaches an internal temperature of 165 degrees with a meat thermometer.

Per serving (with skin): Kcalories 329 (From Fat 122); Fat 14g (Saturated 4g); Cholesterol 125mg; Sodium 589mg; Carbohydrate 1g (Dietary Fiber 0g); Protein 48g.

Tip: Use this easy dry rub on any poultry you like. It's great with chicken, Cornish game hens, capons, and game birds.

Turkey Loaf with Portobello Sauce

Prep time: 25 min • **Cook time:** 1 hr • **Yield:** 4 servings

Ingredients	Directions

The meatloaf:

Nonstick cooking spray

1 medium onion, minced

1 stalk celery, minced

1 pound lean ground turkey

¼ cup chopped parsley

¼ cup fine bread crumbs

¼ cup skim milk

1 egg white, lightly beaten

1 clove garlic, minced

1 teaspoon dried thyme leaves

¼ teaspoon nutmeg

¼ teaspoon pepper

The sauce:

2 teaspoons unsalted margarine

1 large portobello mushroom, cleaned and cut into small pieces (about 1 cup)

1 cup low-sodium chicken broth

⅛ teaspoon ground nutmeg

⅛ teaspoon pepper

⅛ teaspoon salt

1 Preheat the oven to 350 degrees.

2 For the meatloaf, coat a large skillet with cooking spray and place over medium heat until hot. Add the onion and celery. Sauté, stirring often, until translucent, about 5 minutes.

3 Meanwhile, in a large bowl, combine the turkey, parsley, bread crumbs, milk, egg white, garlic, thyme, nutmeg, and pepper. Add the onion and celery and mix well. Form into a loaf and place in a well-coated loaf pan. Bake 50 minutes or until the internal temperature is 165 degrees.

4 For the sauce, melt the margarine in a saucepan placed over medium heat. Add the mushrooms. Sauté, stirring, until tender.

5 Remove from the heat. Add the chicken broth, nutmeg, pepper, and salt. Return to heat. Cook until fragrant and slightly thickened, 5 minutes.

6 When the meatloaf is cooked, unmold, slice, and place portions on warmed dinner plates. Ladle mushroom sauce over sliced turkey loaf.

Per serving: Kcalories 203 (From Fat 32); Fat 4g (Saturated 1g); Cholesterol 76mg; Sodium 243mg; Carbohydrate 11g (Dietary Fiber 2g); Protein 31g.

Turkey Zucchini Burgers

Prep time: 15 min • **Cook time:** 8 min • **Yield:** 6 servings

Ingredients	Directions
1 pound 93 percent lean ground turkey	*1* Preheat the oven to 400 degrees.
2 cups grated zucchini (1 large zucchini)	*2* In a large bowl, combine all the ingredients except the oil and mix well. Shape into 18 small burgers, each about 3 bites.
2 tablespoons parsley	
1 teaspoon cumin	*3* In a large skillet, heat the oil until hot.
2 cloves crushed garlic	
¼ cup chopped red onion	*4* Place the burgers in the skillet and cook on high, browning both sides about 4 minutes until cooked.
1 egg	
2 tablespoons oregano	*5* Transfer the burgers to a baking sheet and bake for 8 minutes.
5 tablespoons canola oil	

Per serving: Kcalories 239 (From Fat 171); Fat 19g (Saturated 3g); Cholesterol 76mg; Sodium 243mg; Carbohydrate 11g (Dietary Fiber 2g); Protein 31g.

Chapter 14

Eating Meat Occasionally

Most of the recipes in this book emphasize the Mediterranean diet. This diet limits red meat to no more than a few times a month. But some people still want to get their red meat fix. So, in this chapter, we include some of the better ways to do that. If you're going to eat red meat, it might as well be delicious!

Protein is an ideal food for people with diabetes because it contains only minimal carbohydrate and, consequently, it doesn't raise blood glucose levels significantly under normal circumstances. Every time you eat, you need to be sure to include some protein to balance the fat and carbohydrate in your diet. Meals that contain protein, as well as fat and starch, help stabilize blood glucose and can give you a more consistent supply of energy. Your body uses protein to build and repair tissues.

In this chapter, we show you three great techniques for cooking meats to fit in with a diabetic diet: searing, braising, and roasting. We give you great recipes for each technique and other tips along the way.

Always cook meats to a safe temperature for appropriate degree of doneness. Consult the following table to find out what temperature to cook the meat of your choice.

Product	Temperature (in degrees)
Ground veal, beef, lamb, pork	160
Beef, medium rare	145
Beef, medium	160
Beef, well done	170
Veal, medium rare	145
Veal, medium	160
Veal, well done	170
Lamb, medium rare	145
Lamb, medium	160
Lamb, well done	170
Pork, medium rare	145
Pork, medium	160
Pork, well done	170
Ham, fresh (raw)	160
Ham, precooked (to reheat)	140

Searing Meats for Culinary Success

A cooking technique called searing is particularly helpful for keeping meat as lowfat and delicious as possible. *Searing* subjects meat to extremely high heat on the stovetop for a short period of time. Usually you sear one side and then the other. The technique produces a beautifully caramelized skin on the meat and essentially seals in its juices. This process helps to retain the moisture content of the meat and therefore much of the flavor.

Veal tenderloin is a healthy option compared with many other cuts of meat that can be quite high in saturated fat and cholesterol. Because it's naturally low in fat, cook veal quickly at high temperatures to keep as many of the natural juices as possible. Searing veal is a great choice.

Veal Tenderloin with Chanterelle Mushrooms in a Muscat Veal Reduction Sauce

Prep time: 15 min • **Cook time:** 15 min • **Yield:** 4 servings

Ingredients	Directions
1 tablespoon cracked black pepper (plus more to taste)	**1** Press ½ teaspoon black pepper into each veal medallion and dredge in the flour.
4 veal tenderloin medallions, approximately 6 ounces each (silver skin removed), pounded thin (check out Chapter 13 for details on pounding meat into cutlets)	**2** Heat a medium sauté pan over high heat. Add olive oil; sear the medallions on both sides (about 4 minutes on each side). Remove the medallions and set aside.
½ cup flour	**3** To the same sauté pan, add the mushrooms, Muscat, salt, remaining 1 teaspoon pepper, and veal stock and cook for 2 minutes over high heat. Adjust salt and pepper to taste. Pour the mixture over the veal slices.
2 tablespoons extra-virgin olive oil	
4 ounces wild mushrooms (chanterelle if available)	
2 ounces Muscat wine	
Salt to taste	
6 ounces veal reduction sauce (reduced veal stock, also known as demi-glace)	

Per serving: Kcalories 424 (From Fat 217); Fat 24g (Saturated 8g); Cholesterol 111mg; Sodium 471mg; Carbohydrate 18g (Dietary Fiber 1g); Protein 32g.

Tip: If you sear a thicker piece of meat like a chop or even a roast, quickly sear the outside and then *finish* the meat in the oven. Searing seals in the natural juices, and roasting finishes the cooking process to desired perfection. Check out Table 14-1, earlier in this chapter, for tips on choosing the right temperature for your taste and your cut of meat.

Tip: If you can't find veal reduction sauce in your grocery store, check online or at Williams-Sonoma.

Pan-Roasted Veal Chops with Corn and Gouda Ragoût

Prep time: 1 hr 15 min • **Cook time:** 45 min • **Yield:** 4 servings

Ingredients	Directions
Steak seasoning:	*1* To prepare the steak seasoning, preheat the oven to 250 degrees. Place the salt, pepper, garlic, and sage into a food processor and process 15 seconds. Transfer to an oven-safe dish and place in the oven for 30 minutes. After the garlic dries out, transfer back to the food processor and process 15 seconds. Set the seasoning aside. Increase the oven temperature to 400 degrees.
1 teaspoon kosher salt	
1 tablespoon cracked black pepper	
1 tablespoon minced garlic	
1 tablespoon chopped fresh sage	
Corn ragoût:	*2* To make the ragoût: Heat a cast-iron skillet over high heat, at least 5 to 6 minutes. Add the corn and continue to cook until it becomes charred, approximately 8 to 10 minutes. Add the garlic, milk, scallions, and pepper. Cook for 2 minutes. Salt and pepper to taste. Reserve.
2 cups yellow corn kernels, fresh or frozen	
½ tablespoon minced garlic	
1 cup milk	
1 tablespoon chopped scallions	
½ teaspoon pepper	*3* Heat a large ovenproof sauté pan over high heat. Season the veal chops with the prepared steak seasoning. Add the olive oil to the heated skillet. Sear the chops in the olive oil until golden brown on both sides, approximately 4 minutes per side. Transfer to the 400-degree oven and roast until desired doneness. Check out Table 14-1 to find the right temperature for you and test your chops with a meat thermometer.
Salt and pepper	
¼ cup grated Gouda cheese	
Veal chops:	*4* When ready to serve, place the corn ragoût on plates and sprinkle the Gouda cheese over the corn. Place the veal chops on top of the corn and serve.
4 veal chops, 7 ounces each	
2 tablespoons steak seasoning (see Step 1)	
2 tablespoons olive oil	

Per serving: Kcalories 351 (From Fat 162); Fat 18g (Saturated 5g); Cholesterol 104mg; Sodium 764mg; Carbohydrate 19g (Dietary Fiber 3g); Protein 30g.

Understanding the Basics of Braising

Braising is a terrific cooking method for meats, vegetables, and anything else you want to make tender and tasty. Basically, *braising* involves cooking a cut of meat in a small amount of liquid. The meat gently cooks and steams, or *braises,* at the same time. Braising is particularly effective for less expensive cuts of meat, because you cook it slowly and break down the tougher muscle over time.

Braising is also a great cooking method because it requires very little use of added fats, such as butter and oil. You can braise foods either in the oven or in a pot on the stove.

Beer-Braised Pork and Crisp-Herb Cabbage with Apple-Tarragon Dipping Sauce

Prep time: 1 hr 45 min • **Cook time:** 1 hr • **Yield:** 6 servings

Ingredients	Directions
¼ teaspoon kosher salt ¼ tablespoon black pepper 4 tablespoons low-sodium soy sauce 2 tablespoons minced shallots 1 tablespoon chopped garlic 1 tablespoon Dijon mustard 1 tablespoon melted butter 2¼ cups amber beer 2½ tablespoons canola oil 1 pound pork tenderloin sliced into 12 1-inch medallions 1 red bell pepper, julienned	*1* Combine the kosher salt, pepper, soy sauce, shallots, garlic, mustard, butter, and beer. Marinate the pork in this mixture in a resealable plastic bag in the refrigerator for 30 to 60 minutes prior to cooking. *2* Heat the oil in a medium-hot large sauté pan. Add the pork medallions, reserving the marinade, and cook until golden brown, about 3 to 4 minutes on each side. *3* Reduce the heat to medium-low and add the reserved marinade and the red bell pepper. Simmer on low, uncovered, for 25 to 30 minutes. Sauce should be reduced by one-half. *4* To serve, place the cabbage (see the next recipe) on a warm plate. Place 2 pork medallions next to the mound of cabbage. Pour the dipping sauce (see the accompanying recipe) into a ramekin and place it next to the pork and cabbage.

Crisp-Herb Cabbage

1 head cabbage, thinly shredded 1 medium red onion, julienned ½ tablespoon chopped garlic (about 2 cloves) ½ cup chopped parsley ¼ cup chopped fresh basil	*1* Combine the cabbage, onion, garlic, parsley, basil, and thyme in a large mixing bowl. *2* Combine the rice vinegar and white vinegar in a small bowl. Add to the cabbage mixture.

1½ teaspoons chopped fresh thyme

½ cup rice vinegar (seasoned)

¼ cup white vinegar

1 tablespoon kosher salt

½ tablespoon crushed red pepper flakes

2 packets Splenda

½ teaspoon allspice

½ teaspoon ground coriander

Juice from 2 lemons

3 Add the salt, red pepper flakes, Splenda, allspice, coriander, and lemon juice to the bowl and mix ingredients well.

4 Let stand at room temperature 45 minutes while getting the other ingredients together.

Apple-Tarragon Dipping Sauce

1 cup water

½ cup rice vinegar

Juice of 1 lemon

2 peeled and diced Granny Smith apples

1 teaspoon chopped garlic

1 bay leaf

¼ teaspoon ground cinnamon

¼ teaspoon ground allspice

½ teaspoon crushed red pepper flakes

1 tablespoon chopped tarragon

Combine all the dipping sauce ingredients in a medium saucepan and bring to a boil. Simmer 20 to 25 minutes, until the apples are tender. Remove the bay leaf. Puree in a food processor until smooth, approximately 3 to 4 minutes.

Per serving (pork, cabbage, and dipping sauce): Kcalories 284 (From Fat 103); Fat 12g (Saturated 3g); Cholesterol 47mg; Sodium 1,946mg; Carbohydrate 29g (Dietary Fiber 6g); Protein 19g.

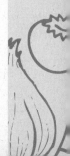

Grilling: Another Healthy Alternative

Grilling is another way to prepare meat and other foods with lots of health benefits. Here are just a few reasons why:

- ✔ As you grill, the fat in the meat drips away, leaving you with leaner meat.

- ✔ The high heat of the grill seals in the moisture in the meat, leaving it more tender. You won't have to add butter or oil.

- ✔ Grilling vegetables along with the meat keeps more vitamins and minerals in the vegetables.

- ✔ Grilled meat retains B vitamins that might be destroyed by other cooking methods.

- ✔ Grilled meats will have a lower calorie content than fried meats.

- ✔ Grilling can be a timesaver because foods generally cook faster on the grill.

 There is some concern that grilling meat may lead to the production of chemicals (called heterocyclic amines and polycyclic hydrocarbons) in the meat that promote cancer. This occurs when the meat is grilled for a long time at very high heat. There are a number of ways to prevent the production of these harmful chemicals:

- ✔ **You can marinate your meat, especially with marinades that contain rosemary.** This has been shown to reduce harmful chemicals by 80 percent.

- ✔ **You can trim the fat before grilling.**

- ✔ **Because steam promotes formation of these chemicals, place tin foil with some holes between the flame and the meat.** The fat will drip through and the foil will reduce the steam.

- ✔ **You can use small cuts of meat that will grill rapidly to reduce the time on the grill.**

- ✔ **Clean the grill thoroughly.** Cleaning the grill will eliminate a source of these chemicals.

- ✔ **If you find that some of the meat is charred, don't eat that part.**

Turkish Meatball Kofte

Prep time: 15 min • **Cook time:** 10 min • **Yield:** 4 servings

Ingredients	Directions
1 pound regular ground lamb	*1* In a large bowl, mix all the ingredients using your hands.
¼ cup breadcrumbs	
1 egg	*2* Make a ball and throw the ball into the bowl 4 or 5 times. (This is a very old technique for bringing all the ingredients together.)
1 onion, grated	
¼ cup fresh parsley, chopped	
½ teaspoon cumin	*3* Divide the large ball into 12 small balls, flatten them into patties, and grill over medium heat for 3 minutes on each side. A little Aioli or tomato sauce on top makes them truly delicious.
1 to 2 garlic cloves, minced	
1 teaspoon salt	
1 teaspoon pepper	

Per serving: Kcalories 300 (From Fat 144); Fat 16g (Saturated 7g); Cholesterol 83mg; Sodium 78mg; Carbohydrate 14g (Dietary Fiber 1g); Protein 22g.

Recommending Roasting

Roasting is a simple technique that requires little effort. Season meat with herbs and spices and cook it in the oven until it reaches a desired degree of doneness. You just need to ensure that the meat doesn't dry out, a possibility with this dry-heat method of cooking. Here are some suggestions:

✔ Slow-roast meat at a low temperature, 350 degrees and below.

✔ Wrap meat in foil for most of the cooking time and remove only for the last half hour of cooking — to allow the meat to brown.

✔ Cook roasts with the bone still attached, when possible, because the meat cooks faster and has more flavor that way.

Try roasting lamb with the next recipe. Leave the bones on the chops for quicker cooking and a beautiful presentation.

Roasted Lamb Sirloin with Herbes de Provence, Spinach, and Onion Ragoût with Lamb Au Jus

Prep time: 45 min • **Cook time:** 1 hr • **Yield:** 4 servings

Ingredients	Directions
4 lamb sirloin chops, 6 ounces each	*1* Preheat the oven to 400 degrees.
2 tablespoons Dijon mustard	*2* Place the lamb sirloin chops in a roasting pan. Spread the Dijon mustard evenly over the lamb chops. Sprinkle on herbes de Provence and lightly salt and pepper. Drizzle lightly with 1 tablespoon of the olive oil and roast 15 minutes. Reduce the heat to 325 degrees and continue roasting until the chops are medium rare (light pink inside), or when a meat thermometer inserted in the center of a chop reaches 145 degrees.
¼ cup herbes de Provence	
Salt and pepper	
2 tablespoons olive oil, divided	
3 white onions, sliced	
2 cups water	*3* While the chops are cooking, combine the onions and water in a large sauté pan or 3-quart saucepan. Cover and simmer until the onions become soft. Remove the onions from the pan and process them in a food processor until they're smooth.
1 bunch spinach	
½ cup port wine	
1 tablespoon chopped garlic	
2 tablespoons butter	*4* In the same sauté pan, heat the remaining olive oil. Add the spinach. Cover and cook the spinach for about 3 to 4 minutes. Fold the onion puree into the spinach, season it lightly with salt and pepper, and set it aside, but keep warm.
	5 Remove the chops from the roasting pan to another dish and cover them with foil to keep them warm.

6 Place the baking pan on the stove. On low heat, deglaze the pan by adding the port wine, garlic, and butter. Reduce the mixture by one-fourth.

7 To serve, place the spinach mixture in the middle of each plate. Place one lamb chop on top of the spinach and pour the port wine sauce over it.

Per serving: Kcalories 281 (From Fat 124); Fat 14g (Saturated 6g); Cholesterol 84mg; Sodium 460mg; Carbohydrate 15g (Dietary Fiber 6g); Protein 26g.

Chapter 15

Snacking without Guilt

In This Chapter

▶ Looking at handy snack options

▶ Using dips and sauces in snacks

▶ Munching on mini-meals

Recipes in This Chapter

↻ Tante Marie's Muesli

↻ Roasted Veggie Dip

↻ Wolfe's BBQ Sauce

▶ Greek-Style Chicken Wraps

▶ Quick Chicken Tostadas

▶ Tuna Dijon Brochettes

↻ Spinach-Ricotta Gnocchi

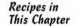

*H*ow many times have you heard, "It's all about portion control"? Well, in this case, the conventional wisdom is true. If your blood glucose levels benefit from a steady stream of food, portion control and snacking are your new best friends. Consider a snack before or after a workout to give you an energy boost. Plan on having a light bite between lunch and dinner. Just keep track of it all and make sure your eating plan is well rounded.

Any food that's part of your healthy daily regimen can be a good snack choice, especially in the right portion sizes. Here's a list of good snack choices for diabetics:

✔ A piece of string cheese and 4 whole-wheat crackers

✔ 8 dried apricot halves

✔ ¾ cup oatmeal (not the sugary just-add-water variety)

✔ Handful of roasted soy nuts

✔ 6 smoked almonds

✔ ½ cup tuna, light mayo, and dill pickle relish

✔ 6 ounces vegetable juice

✔ ½ cup cottage cheese

Watch out for snacks from vending machines and prepackaged foods like pudding cups, instant flavored oatmeal, and toaster pastries. Although they can be convenient, they can also be loaded with sugar, salt, and fat. Read your labels carefully before making your food choices. For more on reading food nutrition labels as a diabetic, check out Chapter 5.

In this chapter, we show you how to stock up on handy snacks, supplement snacks with dips and sauces, and whip up light and easy mini-meals.

Keeping Healthy Snacks at the Ready

Many people grab whatever they can find for a quick snack because they're incredibly hungry. It's easy to reach for a bag of chips, a candy bar, or a soda if they're handy. Instead of keeping these convenient, high-fat, high-sodium, high-sugar foods handy, stock your fridge, freezer, and pantry with healthy snacks that can satisfy you and keep you eating on your plan. For example, you can make snack-size servings of cut-up fresh veggies, ready and waiting in the fridge.

For a special beverage treat, keep some sugar-free drink mix single-serving tubes handy. Just add their contents to your water bottle for an instant treat.

Mixing it up with whole grains

Stock your pantry today with healthy whole-grain snacks like GORP. Here we include whole grains, nuts, and dried fruit for a good all-around snack choice. Feel free to substitute your favorite fruits and nuts as you experiment with this tasty treat.

Tante Marie's Muesli

Prep time: 10 min • **Yield:** 6 servings

Ingredients	Directions
3 cups rolled oats (regular, not instant)	**1** Place all the ingredients in a large bowl, and mix well.
½ cup bran	**2** Store in an airtight container in your pantry for up to one week.
½ cup wheat germ	
1 cup raisins	
1 cup chopped dried apples	
½ cup toasted hazelnuts and/or almonds (no salt added)	
2 tablespooons brown sugar (not packed)	

Per serving: Kcalories 387 (Calories from Fat 87); Fat 10g (Saturated 1g); Cholesterol 0mg; Sodium 23 mg; Carbohydrate 69g (Dietary Fiber 12g); Protein 12g.

Tip: If you prefer your oats toasted, place the rolled oats on a baking sheet in an oven preheated to 350 degrees for about 15 minutes, stirring from time to time.

Vary It! You can substitute rolled wheat and/or rye flakes for oats.

Tip: Muesli can be served softened with yogurt and served with fresh fruit as they do in Switzerland, or served with milk.

Why should you choose whole-grain snacks?

If you can have 6 saltines or 4 whole-wheat crackers and you're really hungry, which should you choose? At first glance, the answer may seem obvious. Choose the saltines because you get 6 (compared to the 4 whole-wheat crackers). But believe it or not, 4 whole-wheat crackers will keep you fuller, longer. The whole grain is the key. Your body works harder and longer to digest the whole-wheat crackers. With saltine crackers, the flour manufacturer has done much of the work for you by refining the flour, removing most of the fiber and nutrients. By making your body work for its nutrition, you help it work more efficiently, in turn helping you to stabilize your blood glucose levels. For more about adding grains to your diet, check out Chapter 10.

Filling your freezer with treats

Some people just can't seem to stay away from the snacks after dinner, especially the sweet ones. Maybe you just want something simple like a bowl of ice cream or a more elegant chocolate mousse or cheesecake. Instead, consider stocking your freezer with the following healthy, quick-grab snacks.

- ✔ **Flavored ice cubes:** Fill ice cube trays with your favorite sugar-free drinks, like any flavor of Crystal Light. Freeze until frozen and then transfer the individual ice cubes to a resealable plastic bag. Add a few lemonade ice cubes to your next glass of strawberry kiwi beverage. Experiment with flavors you like.

- ✔ **Grapes:** Clean the grapes and remove them from their stems. Place individual grapes on a clean baking sheet in the freezer. When the grapes are frozen, transfer them to a resealable plastic bag. Grab a few when your sweet tooth attacks.

- ✔ **Sugar-free frozen pops:** Many manufacturers are making freezer pops from 100 percent juice or sweetening them with sugar substitutes.

- ✔ **Yogurt tubes:** Squeezable yogurt tubes can make a terrific quick snack. Toss a few in the freezer for an extra creamy frozen treat.

This type of yogurt can have added sugar, so read your labels carefully to make sure you know what you're eating, and confirm that it fits with your eating goals.

Choosing kid-friendly snacks

Many children are afflicted by diabetes. Often, their parents and other caregivers need to learn about the disease from scratch. Check out Chapter 22 for more tips on helping kids cope with diabetes. Also, check out *Diabetes For Dummies,* 4th Edition, written by Alan L. Rubin, MD, and published by Wiley, for more great kid-friendly tips.

Here's a list of snacks designed with diabetic kids in mind. Teach kids how to snack well early in life, and they'll be better equipped to deal with diabetes as they grow.

- Snack-sized bag of light microwave popcorn
- Whole-wheat pretzels with mustard
- Cup of lowfat yogurt
- Sugar-free gelatin cup
- Lunchmeat rollup
- An apple with a small dollop of peanut butter
- Celery sticks dipped in lowfat ranch dressing
- Turkey hot dog
- ½ cup cottage cheese
- 1 ounce part-skim string cheese
- ¼ cup roasted peanuts

Adding Dips and Sauces to Snacks

Condiments are typically used to flavor or complement other foods. But some condiments are so delicious and desirable that you may want to eat them all by themselves. *Condiment* may be a bit of an understatement for the tasty recipes in this section. They can both be terrific spreads for sandwiches or lettuce wraps. Use them as sauces to top grilled chicken or firm fish.

Dips are a creative way to get in lots of vegetables. Unfortunately, most dips tend to be very high in calories and fat. What is considered a light snack can quickly turn into a full meal's worth of calories and fat. So skip the fat and keep the flavor with this excellent vegetable dip. (Check out Chapter 7 for more dips to try.)

Roasted Veggie Dip

Prep time: 20 min • **Cook time:** 35 min • **Yield:** 6 servings

Ingredients	*Directions*
½ eggplant, peeled, thick sliced	*1* Preheat the oven to 400 degrees. Spray the eggplant, zucchini, squash, onion, and garlic with the cooking spray, coating well.
1 zucchini, thick sliced	
1 yellow squash, thick sliced	*2* In a small bowl, combine the cayenne pepper, seasoning salt, and chili powder. Add one-fourth of the seasoning to the vegetables. Toss well to combine. Add another one-fourth of the seasoning and toss well. Repeat until the vegetables are evenly coated and all the seasoning is added. Adding the seasonings in stages helps combine the seasonings evenly.
½ red onion, thick sliced	
4 cloves garlic, roughly chopped	
Nonstick cooking spray	
½ teaspoon cayenne pepper	
1 teaspoon seasoning salt	*3* Spray a baking pan with the cooking spray. Add the vegetables in a single layer. Cook vegetables in the oven, until browned, stirring occasionally, roughly 35 minutes.
1 teaspoon chili powder	
Salt and pepper	
	4 Place the roasted veggies in the bowl of a food processor. Process to desired consistency. Season with salt and pepper as necessary.

Per serving: Kcalories 32 (From Fat 3); Fat 0g (Saturated 0g); Cholesterol 0mg; Sodium 257mg; Carbohydrate 7g (Dietary Fiber 3g); Protein 2g.

Wolfe's BBQ Sauce

Prep time: 10 min • **Cook time:** 15 min • **Yield:** 8 servings

Ingredients	Directions
1½ cups ketchup	Place all ingredients in a nonmetallic saucepan on low. Warm the sauce for 10 minutes, stirring occasionally. For thicker sauce, continue to cook for 2 to 3 more minutes. Remove from the heat and cool.
1 cup light pancake syrup	
1½ tablespoons low-sodium soy sauce	
1½ tablespoons Worcestershire sauce	
¾ tablespoon sesame oil	
1 teaspoon minced ginger	
1 teaspoon chili powder	
1 teaspoon onion powder	
1 teaspoon fresh chopped garlic	
1 teaspoon pepper	
½ teaspoon salt	

Per serving: Kcalories 131 (From Fat 29); Fat 3g (Saturated 1g); Cholesterol 0mg; Sodium 872mg; Carbohydrate 26g (Dietary Fiber 1g); Protein 1g.

Preparing Mini-Meals

Eating small portions of well-balanced meals can be a great way to fit a nutritious and filling snack into your day. Maybe you ate a light brunch and are waiting for a late dinner. Maybe you had a really early breakfast and can't fit a full lunch in until late in the day. Or maybe you just find it easier to maintain even blood sugar levels by eating five or six small meals each day. Whatever the reason, mini-meals can help you eat right.

Choosing chicken

For diabetics, chicken is a great basis for a mini-meal because it provides protein that is slowly changed to sugar in your body. Try the following two recipes to enjoy a taste of chicken.

Greek-Style Chicken Wraps

Prep time: 20 min • **Cook time:** 25 min • **Yield:** 2 servings

Ingredients	Directions
Nonstick cooking spray	**1** Preheat the oven to 350 degrees. Coat an 8 x 8 inch baking dish with nonstick cooking spray. Brush the chicken breast on both sides with lemon juice and oregano. Place the chicken breast and onion in the baking dish. Bake for approximately 25 minutes.
2 boneless, skinless chicken breasts, 4 ounces each, pounded thin	
1 tablespoon lemon juice	
1 teaspoon oregano, crushed and dried	**2** When the chicken is done, transfer to a cutting board and cut into ½-inch strips.
2 thin slices Vidalia onion	
2 whole-wheat tortillas, 10-inch variety	**3** Spread out the tortillas on a flat surface. Spread equal parts of yogurt on top of the tortillas. Top with equal parts chicken, onion, cucumber, cheese, and mint.
¼ cup lowfat plain yogurt	
¼ cup peeled, seeded, and chopped cucumber	**4** Roll up the wraps and serve warm.
¼ cup crumbled feta cheese	
1 teaspoon chopped fresh mint	

Per serving: Kcalories 372 (From Fat 97); Fat 11g (Saturated 4g); Cholesterol 81mg; Sodium 767mg; Carbohydrate 36g (Dietary Fiber 7g); Protein 33g.

Quick Chicken Tostadas

Prep time: 20 min • **Cook time:** 10 min • **Yield:** 6 servings

Ingredients	*Directions*
6 whole-wheat flour tortillas Nonstick cooking spray ¾ pound cooked chicken (see the tip at the end of the recipe) ¾ cup salsa ¼ teaspoon cayenne pepper ¼ teaspoon chili powder 1 cup diced red bell pepper Salt and pepper	*1* Preheat the oven to 400 degrees. Spray each tortilla lightly with cooking spray. Place prepared tortillas on a baking sheet and place in the oven. Toast the tortillas until crisp, approximately 2 to 3 minutes. Remove from the oven and set aside. Reduce the oven temperature to 375 degrees.
	2 Mix the chicken, salsa, cayenne pepper, chili powder, red bell pepper, and salt and pepper to taste together in a mixing bowl. Top each tostada with one-sixth of the chicken mixture.
1 cup shredded cheddar cheese 1 tablespoon minced cilantro or green onions (optional) 2 tablespoons minced black olives (optional) 6 tablespoons lowfat sour cream (optional) 3 tablespoons prepared gua-camole (optional)	*3* For each tostada, top the chicken mixture with one-sixth of the cheddar cheese. Return the tostadas to the oven. Cook until the chicken is heated through and the cheese is melted, approximately 5 to 7 minutes.
	4 If desired, top each tostada with ½ teaspoon cilantro or green onions, 1 tablespoon sour cream, and 1 teaspoon black olives.

Per serving: Kcalories 316 (From Fat 121); Fat 13g (Saturated 5g); Cholesterol 68mg; Sodium 668mg; Carbohydrate 31g (Dietary Fiber 2g); Protein 29g.

Tip: For this recipe, you can purchase roasted chicken breast, or you can cook the chicken breast yourself by poaching it, which means cooking it in water just below the boiling point until it is cooked through (no longer pink inside).

Selecting seafood

Seafood, tuna in particular, is a great item for a diabetic to choose as a mini-meal because, like chicken, it's mostly protein and does not raise your sugar rapidly. The following dish is easy to reduce to a snack size portion: Eat only one skewer full of tasty goodness, and you cut the kilocalories (and the other nutritional analysis) in half. Enjoy!

Tuna Dijon Brochettes

Prep time: 25 min • **Cook time:** 6–8 min • **Yield:** 1 serving

Ingredients	Directions
8 ounces tuna, fresh, cut into 6 equal chunks	**1** Preheat the broiler. In a bowl, coat the tuna chunks with the mustard.
1 tablespoon Dijon mustard	
4 mushrooms	**2** Using 2 metal skewers, each 8 inches long, skewer the tuna, mushrooms, peppers, zucchini, pineapple, and cherry tomatoes, alternating each item twice, beginning and ending with a tuna chunk.
4 squares red bell pepper, 1 inch each	
4 slices zucchini, ¼-inch thick	
4 chunks fresh, peeled pineapple, 1 inch each	**3** Sprinkle each skewer with salt and pepper to taste. Coat a baking sheet with the cooking spray and place the skewers on the baking sheet. Broil for 6 to 8 minutes.
4 medium cherry tomatoes	
Salt and pepper	
Nonstick cooking spray	

Per serving: Kcalories 351 (From Fat 40); Fat 4g (Saturated 1g); Cholesterol 98mg; Sodium 762mg; Carbohydrate 23g (Dietary Fiber 5g); Protein 56g.

Stocking your snack drawer at work

Getting through the workday and avoiding food pitfalls can be challenging for anyone, particularly so for the diabetic. The best defense against the shared snacks of coffeecakes, muffins, bagels, and doughnuts near the coffee station is a good offense. Keep a healthy snack drawer at work for snacking emergencies, and you're sure to save yourself some calories and blood sugar spikes and dips. And remember: A well-stocked snack drawer can be a lifesaver on early days when you don't have time to eat breakfast before heading for work.

Here are some ideas for a diabetic's snack drawer:

✓ Light popcorn in snack-sized microwaveable bags

✓ Individual servings of nuts

✓ Lowfat and low-sodium canned soups

✓ Fat-free, sugar-free gelatin and pudding

✓ Low-sugar protein bars

✓ Canned nutritional supplement drinks, like Glucerna or Ensure

✓ Individual servings of sugar-free drink mixes

✓ Individual cans of low-sodium vegetable juice

✓ No-sugar-added juice boxes or bottles

When possible, choose individual serving sizes. They're proportioned to take the brainwork out of grabbing a quick snack when you're starved. Plus, keeping track of how much you eat is much easier when the nutritional information is on each snack.

Picking pasta

Indulge in your cravings for Italian food with this version of the traditional potato pasta, gnocchi. Potatoes, or pasta for that matter, may be tough to work into your eating plan, but if you love Italian food, you don't have to give it up completely. In addition to this great flour-free option, check out Zucchini and Cucumber Linguine with Clams found in Chapter 11. You get all the Italian flavor without any traditional pasta and the costly carbs.

Spinach-Ricotta Gnocchi

Prep time: 1 hr • **Cook time:** 4–5 min • **Yield:** 4 servings

Ingredients	Directions
½ **pound part-skim ricotta cheese**	***1*** Place the ricotta in a strainer lined with cheesecloth and let sit overnight in the refrigerator to remove excess liquid.
1 gallon water	
¼ **pound fresh spinach**	***2*** Bring the 1 gallon of water to a boil, add the spinach, and boil for 30 seconds. Strain the spinach and place the spinach on a baking sheet lined with parchment paper. Place the spinach in the refrigerator to cool. Once cooled, squeeze out all the excess water from the spinach. Chop the spinach as fine as you can on a cutting board. This may take some time, but the finer the better.
1 cup grated Parmesan cheese	
1 egg, beaten	
Pinch ground nutmeg	
Salt to taste	
2 tablespoons potato starch	***3*** To make the gnocchi, place the chopped spinach, ricotta, Parmesan cheese, egg, nutmeg, and a pinch of salt into a large mixing bowl. Mix until the spinach has been evenly distributed, and add the potato starch, dehydrated potato, and 2 tablespoons of the flour to bind the mixture. Bring a small pot of water to a boil and drop a spoon-sized piece of gnocchi to test the consistency and flavor. If the gnocchi is too wet and falls apart, add another egg and some flour. The key to this gnocchi is to add the minimum amount of binder so that the gnocchi are as light as possible.
1 tablespoon dehydrated potato flakes	
2 tablespoons plus 2 cups flour	
	4 Place a 6-quart pot on the stove with plenty of salted water to boil the gnocchi. Bring the water to a boil and turn down until you're ready to cook the gnocchi.
	5 Place the remaining 2 cups of flour in a long baking pan. Shake the flour evenly around in the pan. Place the gnocchi mixture into a pastry bag with a large straight tip about ½ inch in diameter. Pipe the gnocchi mixture in a long line directly into the flour, as if you were making a long snakelike piece. You can make a couple of lines like this in the flour.

6   With a knife, cut the snakelike pieces into 1-inch pieces. With your hands, gently cover the gnocchi lightly with flour, shake off any excess flour, and place directly into boiling salt water. Cook the gnocchi for at least 5 minutes or until they float for 2 minutes. Remove from the water.

Per serving: Kcalories 282 (From Fat 109); Fat 12g (Saturated 7g); Cholesterol 86mg; Sodium 628mg; Carbohydrate 24g (Dietary Fiber 1g); Protein 19g.

Tip: You can serve these immediately or hold them for later use. If you plan to hold the gnocchi, place the cooked gnocchi onto a lightly oiled sheet pan and place in the refrigerator. Once cooled, you can place the gnocchi in an airtight container until ready to use. You can reheat the gnocchi in boiling water for 4 to 5 minutes.

Chapter 16

Making Room for Dessert

In This Chapter

▶ Filling out your meal plans with fruits

▶ Using juices the right way

▶ Exploring agave nectar

▶ Enjoying chocolate treats

Sugar is not a dirty word, even for a diabetic. But it's no secret that the amount of sugar consumed by Americans today is out of control. Manufacturers sneak it into all kinds of products, including prepackaged rice pilaf mix, ketchup, and, of course, baked goods, under the names high-fructose corn syrup and malt syrup. Even though diabetes is a disease that involves impaired metabolism of carbohydrates, you can still enjoy desserts that contain starches and sugar. You just need to select your ingredients wisely and eat reasonably modest portions. But don't waste time feeling guilty because you can't stay away from sweets. Sweet is one of the basic tastes, just like sour and salty, and craving sweet foods is normal.

In this chapter, we show you how to create appealing desserts that feature nutritious ingredients. We help you satisfy your cravings for sweet foods, including chocolate. We introduce a healthful sweetener, agave nectar, to flavor desserts the right way. And we give you a host of different presentations to impress your guests.

Finding a New Take on Fruit

Diabetic desserts have long consisted of sugar-free gelatin and fruit. There's certainly nothing wrong with that, but if you're bored with the standard take on fruit, we have several recipes that help you improve upon that old standard, fruit, and give it an update you'd be proud to serve to anyone.

Spiced Infusion with Tropical Fruits

Prep time: 5 min • **Cook time:** 30 min • **Yield:** 2 servings

Ingredients	*Directions*
¼ cup Splenda for Baking	**1** Combine all the ingredients, except the fruit, in a large saucepan and bring to a boil. Turn off the heat, cover, and allow to steep ½ hour. Strain spices and herbs and allow to cool completely.
2½ cups water	
8 star anise	
2 vanilla beans	**2** Serve on top of the fruit.
2 tablespoons gingerroot	
Zest of 1 lemon	
1 cinnamon stick	
15 whole black peppercorns	
1 teaspoon coriander seed	
1½ cups fresh tropical fruits, such as mango, pineapple, star fruit, or passion fruit	

Per serving (sauce with 4 ounces fruit): Kcalories 199 (From Fat 6); Fat 1g (Saturated 0g); Cholesterol 0mg; Sodium 18mg; Carbohydrate 50g (Dietary Fiber 7g); Protein 2g.

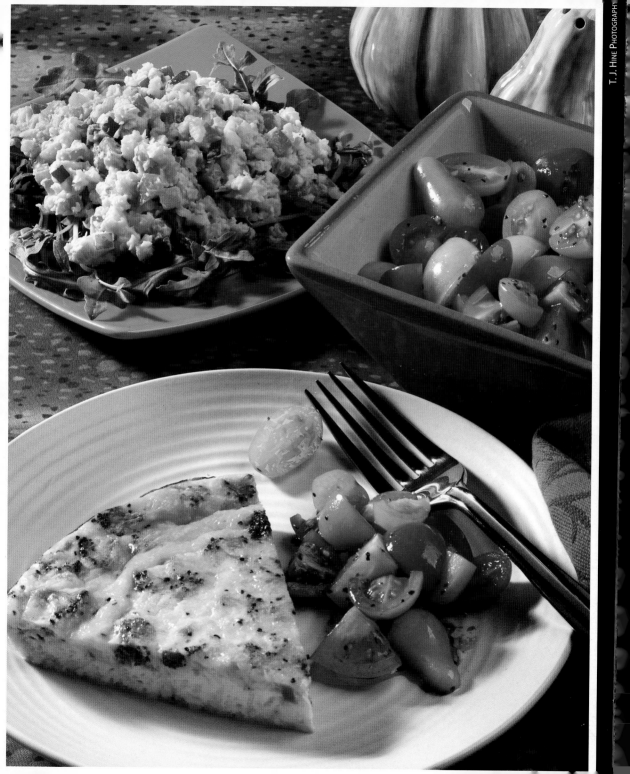

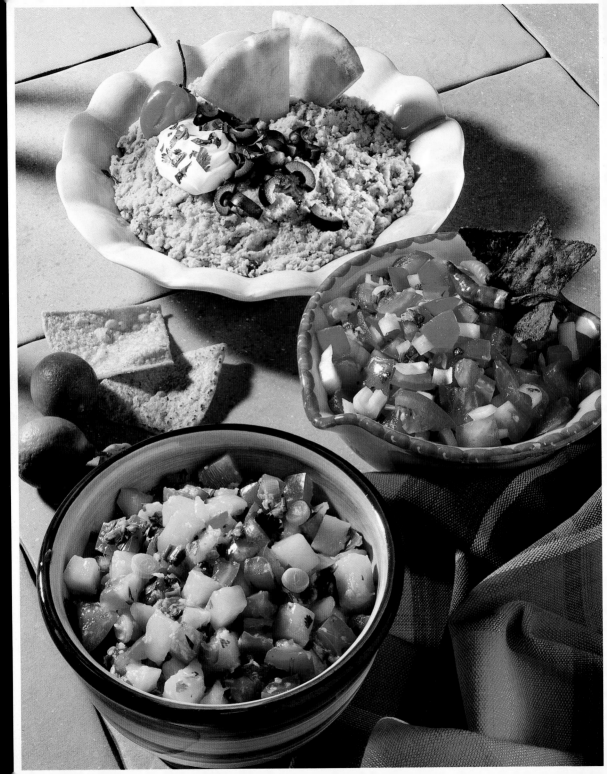

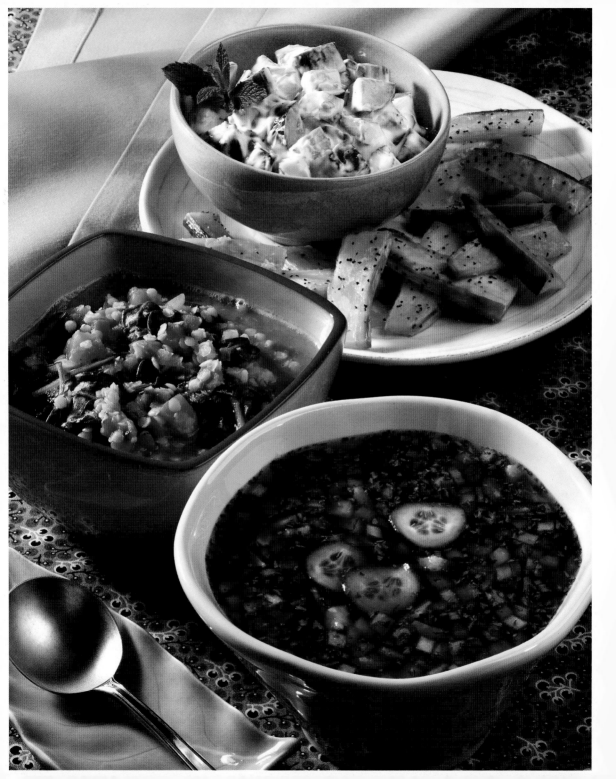

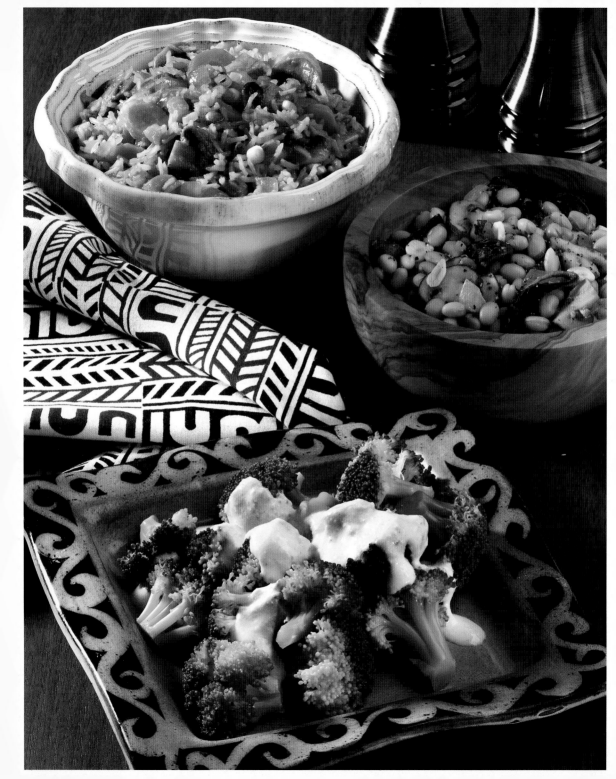

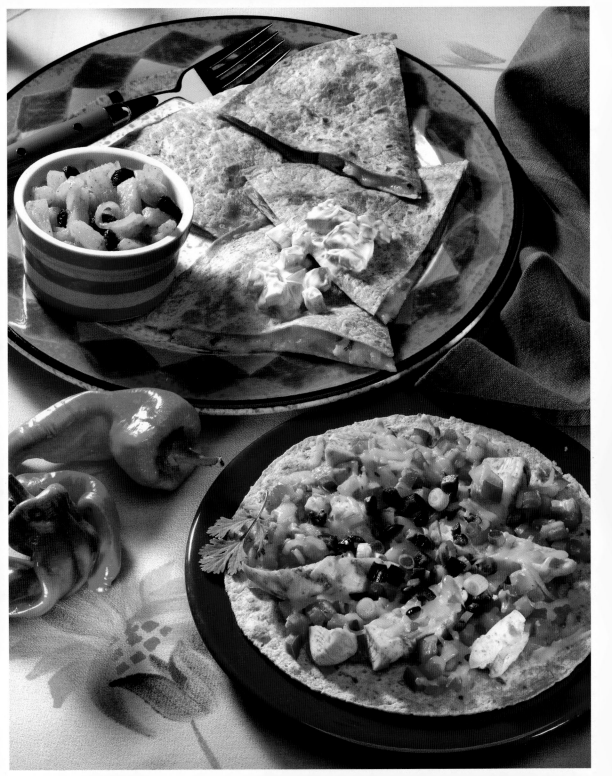

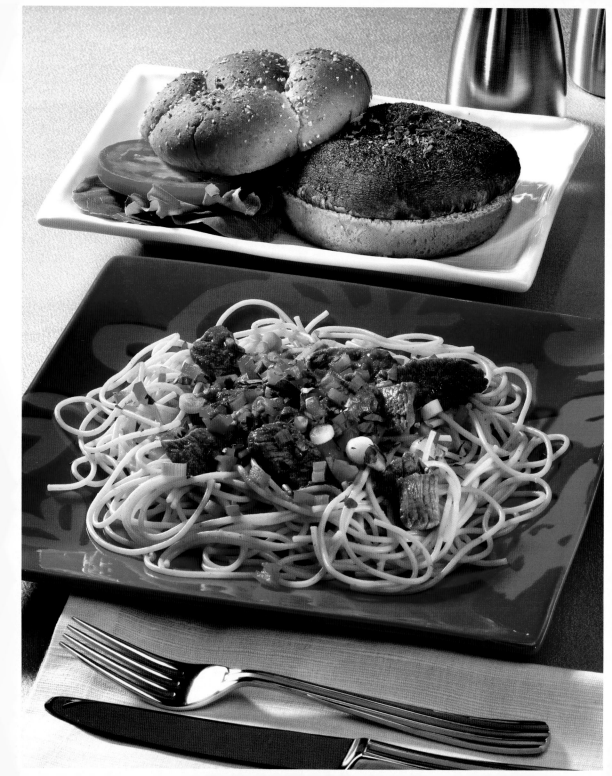

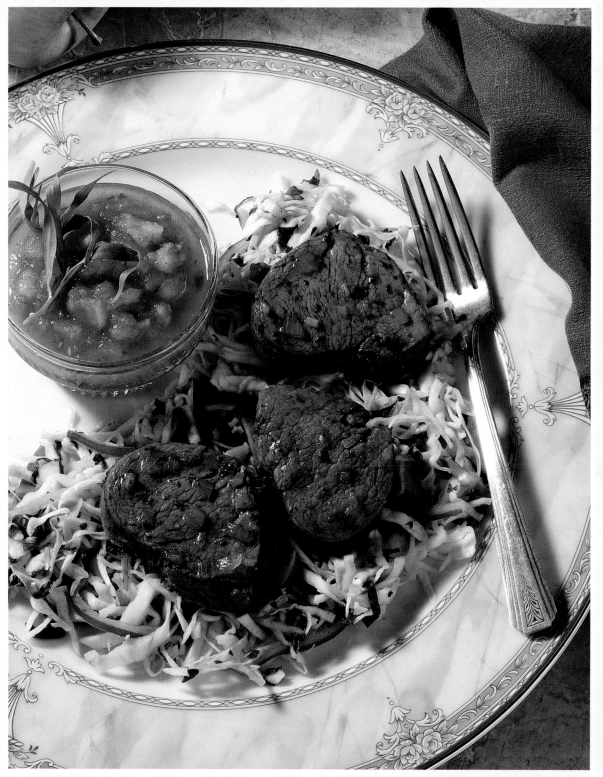

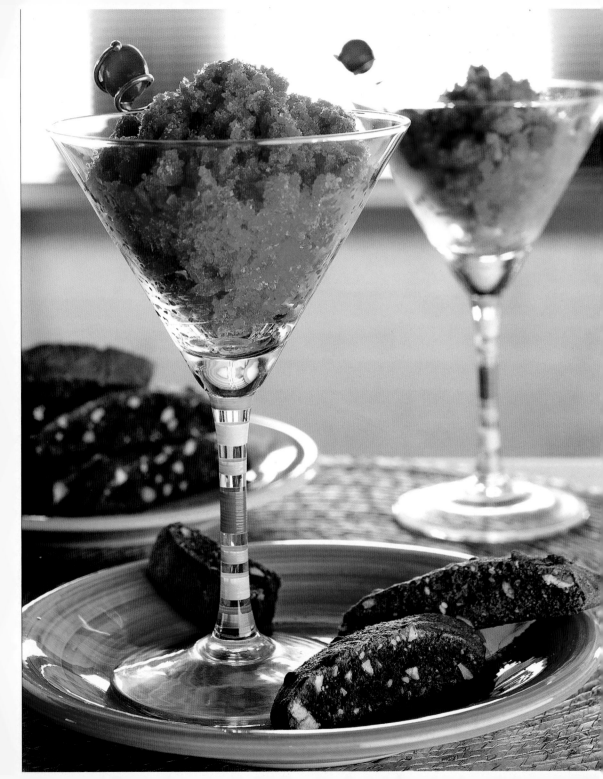

Creating luscious fruit desserts with different flavorings

Even if you don't have time to prepare a full-blown fruit recipe, you can still concoct wonderful desserts and mouthwatering nibbles simply by using luscious fruit and adding a special ingredient or two. You can use all sorts of herbs, spices, and nuts to enhance the flavor of fruit. Some examples include:

✔ Peel a banana, freeze it, and then puree it in a food processor, along with almond or peanut butter, and you'll have a fruit version of ice cream.

✔ Puree ripe melon with lowfat vanilla yogurt, a dash of nutmeg and cinnamon, and a squirt of lemon for a refreshing fruit soup.

✔ Combine brown sugar substitute and lowfat vanilla yogurt. Layer the yogurt with fresh fruit to create a parfait.

✔ Grill pineapple slices and then lightly coat with lemon juice, a dash of honey, and cinnamon.

✔ Create fruit kabobs from your fresh favorites and marinate them in lemon juice, nutmeg, and crushed mint.

One of the easiest ways to spice up a fruit dessert is by adding, well, spices. Try sprinkling fresh fruit with traditional Indian spices like green cardamom or with a Latin-inspired combination of cayenne pepper and cinnamon. Get started with the spiced fruit in the next recipe.

 Ginger and lemon brighten the sweet flavors of the cantaloupe and papaya in the following recipe. Choose cantaloupes that are heavy for their size and have a lightly sweet melon fragrance. A cantaloupe should be firm but give slightly when pressed. Avoid melons with mushy spots or discolorations.

The papaya is a large pear-shaped tropical fruit. It contains a bed of large peppery seeds in the center of the fruit. If you're looking for a ripe papaya to use immediately or refrigerate, choose richly colored papayas, with splotches of bright yellow, green, and some orange. Green papayas will ripen in a few days if left at room temperature and placed in a brown paper bag.

Cantaloupe-Papaya Salad with Ginger Simple Syrup

Prep time: 20 min • **Cook time:** 10 min • **Yield:** 6 servings

Ingredients	Directions
Syrup:	**1** Bring the Splenda and water to a boil in a small saucepan over moderate heat. Add the gingerroot and reduce the heat, allowing the liquid to simmer.
¼ **cup (18 packets) Splenda**	
½ **cup water**	
2 inches fresh gingerroot, peeled	**2** Stir until the Splenda dissolves and the gingerroot infuses the syrup, about 2 minutes. Remove the pan from heat and take out the gingerroot. Allow the syrup to cool at room temperature. Add the lemon zest.
1 tablespoon lemon zest	
Fruit salad:	
1 cantaloupe	**3** Scoop out the meat of the fruits with a melon baller and then toss it with the simple syrup and mint when you're ready to serve it.
2 papayas	
4 mint sprigs	

Per serving: Kcalories 78 (From Fat 1); Fat 0g (Saturated 0g); Cholesterol 0mg; Sodium 20mg; Carbohydrate 19g (Dietary Fiber 3g); Protein 1g.

Pears Baked in Red Wine alla Piemontese

Prep time: 15 min • **Cook time:** 1½ hr • **Yield:** 4 servings

Ingredients	Directions
10 ounces dry red wine **7 cloves** **1 cinnamon stick** **Juice of 2 lemons** **1 cup Splenda** **4 large Bosc pears, unpeeled**	*1* Preheat the oven to 300 degrees. *2* Pour the wine into a 9-inch-square baking pan. Add the cloves, cinnamon, lemon juice, and Splenda and stir until the Splenda dissolves. Add the pears to the pan. Place them in the oven and bake for 1½ hours, brushing the pears with wine from the pan every 10 minutes. The skins should be brown and crinkly when you remove the pears from the oven. *3* Remove the pears from the oven. Allow them to cool at room temperature and serve.

Per serving: Kcalories 160 (From Fat 8); Fat 1g (Saturated 0g); Cholesterol 0mg; Sodium 0mg; Carbohydrate 40g (Dietary Fiber 5g); Protein 1g.

Strawberry-Rhubarb Compote

Prep time: 10 min • **Cook time:** 25 min • **Yield:** 5 servings

Ingredients	Directions
4 cups rhubarb sliced about ½-inch thick 2 cups fresh strawberries, sliced and hulled ¼ cup sugar plus 12 packets sucralose 1 teaspoon cinnamon ¼ cup water	*1* In a large saucepan, combine all the ingredients and bring to a boil. Cook slowly until the rhubarb and strawberries are soft.
	2 Chill until cool and serve.

Per serving: Kcalories 80 (From Fat 0); Fat 0g (Saturated 0g); Cholesterol 0mg; Sodium 5mg; Carbohydrate 20g (Dietary Fiber 3g); Protein 1g.

Vary It! You can vary the taste by adding ginger, vanilla bean, peppermint, or anything you think sounds good!

Juicing Your Way to Tasty and Healthy Treats

Fruit juice lacks the fiber of whole fruit, so all the natural sugars can really affect your blood sugar without all the fiber to slow it down. But with a little diligence, you can use fruit juice to flavor your desserts and still maintain your blood sugar levels.

Cranberry-Raspberry Granita

Prep time: 6 hr 30 min, mostly unattended • **Yield:** 6 servings

Ingredients	Directions
2 cups 100% juice cranberry-raspberry juice blend **1½ cups raspberries (fresh or previously frozen, thawed, and drained)** **½ cup Splenda sugar substitute**	**1** In a blender, combine the juice and raspberries. Mix well. Pour the mixture through a fine-mesh sieve placed over a mixing bowl. Press the mixture gently through the sieve, as necessary, to extract as much juice as possible. Discard the mixture in the sieve or reserve for another use.
	2 Add the Splenda to the strained juice mixture and stir to mix well. Cover and freeze. Stir thoroughly with a fork about every 30 minutes, for 6 hours or so, or until the granita is frozen in a crumbly, grainy texture.

Per serving: Kcalories 71 (From Fat 2); Fat 0g (Saturated 0g); Cholesterol 0mg; Sodium 2mg; Carbohydrate 18g (Dietary Fiber 0g); Protein 0g.

Granita of Lemon

Prep time: 15 min plus freezing • **Yield:** 4 servings

Ingredients	*Directions*
1¼ cups lemon juice, preferably from Meyer lemons	*1* In a medium bowl, place the lemon juice. Set aside.
½ cup sugar **1¾ cup water**	*2* In a saucepan, combine the water and sugar. Make a syrup by heating the mixture until it starts to boil.
	3 Remove from the heat and add to the lemon juice. Stir and let cool for about half an hour.
	4 Pour the mixture into a freezer-proof container. Place flat in the freezer.
	5 Remove from the freezer every hour and whisk to break up the larger ice crystals until all the liquid is frozen.
	6 To serve, scoop frozen granita into old-fashioned glasses. Store covered in the freezer.

Per serving: Kcalories 90 (From Fat 0); Fat 0g (Saturated 0g); Cholesterol 0mg; Sodium 1mg; Carbohydrate 22.5g (Dietary Fiber 0g); Protein 0g.

Tip: Citrus fruits in particular make great juice choices for adding to desserts. Their strong flavors mean a little can go a long way. And many are tart rather than sweet, so they naturally have few sugars. For the scoop on how to juice your own citrus, check out Chapter 7.

Taking Advantage of Agave Nectar

Agave nectar is a delicious natural sweetener with a flavor similar to honey. It's derived from the same plant that gives us tequila. Compared to other sweeteners, it has a low glycemic index. It provides sweetness without the sugar rush (and subsequent crash) of refined sugars. Used in moderation, it can be part of a healthy diabetic diet.

Additionally, agave nectar, sometimes called agave syrup, is full of other health benefits, including improving bacterial balance in the gut. When mixed with salt, it's a beneficial treatment for wound care. Inulin, one of the components of agave, may help lower cholesterol, reduce the risk of some cancers, and improve the absorption of nutrients, like isoflavones, calcium, and magnesium.

Brown Rice Pudding

Prep time: 10 min • **Cook time:** 1 hr 45 min • **Yield:** 6 servings

Ingredients	Directions
1¼ cups brown rice 3 cups soymilk ½ cup golden raisins ½ cup raisins 2 teaspoons agave nectar	**1** Cook rice according to package directions, stirring often.
	2 Combine the cooked rice with the soymilk, raisins, and agave nectar. Cover and cook the mixture over low heat for 1 hour, until most of the soymilk has evaporated and the rice is creamy.

Per serving: Kcalories 288 (Calories from Fat 32); Fat 3g (Saturated 1g); Cholesterol 0mg; Sodium 26mg; Carbohydrate 58g (Dietary Fiber 6g); Protein 8g.

Crispy Oatmeal Cookies

Prep time: 15 min • **Cook time:** 24 min • **Yield:** 12 servings, 2 cookies per serving

Ingredients	Directions
½ **cup grape seed oil**	**1** Preheat oven to 350 degrees.
½ **cup agave nectar**	
¼ **cup soymilk**	**2** Mix grape seed oil, agave nectar, soymilk, and vanilla. Add oats, baking soda, cinnamon, and flours to the liquid mixture. Mix until well combined.
1 teaspoon vanilla extract	
3 cups old-fashioned rolled oats	**3** Using a small spoon, drop dough on nonstick cookie sheet and flatten with wet fingers or spatula, roughly 2 inches apart.
½ **teaspoon baking soda**	
2 teaspoons cinnamon	
½ **cup white flour**	**4** Bake 12 minutes or until golden brown and crispy.
½ **cup whole-wheat flour**	**5** Removed baked cookies from cookie sheet and place on a cooling rack. Allow to cool completely. Store cooled cookies in an airtight container.

Per serving (2 cookies): Kcalories 236 (Calories from Fat 95); Fat 11g (Saturated 1g); Cholesterol 0mg; Sodium 54mg; Carbohydrate 32g (Dietary Fiber 4g); Protein 5g.

Choosing Chocolate for Dessert

What would life be without chocolate? Fortunately, you won't have to speculate or even discover the situation for yourself. Mix up your own tasty chocolate concoctions by substituting your favorite no-calorie sweetener for the regular sugar.

And whenever possible, choose the highest-quality cocoa powder you can afford. The flavor is much better, and since you're only having a small portion anyway, you definitely want the best-tasting bite you can get!

Mixing up some meringues

Meringue, essentially egg whites flavored and whipped to foamy peaks, is an extremely versatile food. You can create little clouds to hold fresh fruit, top a fruit pie, or even use it to cover a pound cake and ice cream (to create baked Alaska). Meringue is naturally lowfat and takes on the flavor of any extracts, like almond, mint, or chocolate, so experiment and enjoy!

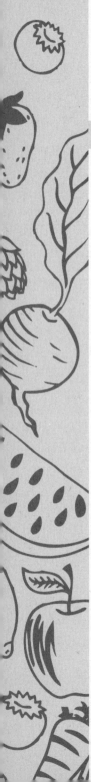

Chocolate Meringue Bits with Strawberries and Cream

Prep time: 30 min, plus standing time of 8 hr • **Cook time:** 1 hr 30 min • **Yield:** 40 1½-inch meringues

Ingredients	Directions
4 egg whites	**1** Preheat the oven to 225 degrees. Line 2 baking sheets with parchment paper.
¼ teaspoon cream of tartar	
1 teaspoon vanilla extract	**2** Beat the egg whites, cream of tartar, and vanilla at high speed with an electric mixer until frothy. Add the Splenda, 1 tablespoon at a time, beating until stiff peaks form, roughly 5 to 7 minutes. Gently fold in the cocoa powder until completely incorporated.
⅔ cup Splenda	
⅓ cup cocoa powder	
1 cup reduced-fat tub-style whipped topping	
40 strawberries	**3** Spoon heaping tablespoons of the mixture onto the baking sheets. Bake for 1 hour and 30 minutes; turn the oven off. Let the meringues stand in the closed oven for 8 hours or overnight. Store in an airtight container.
	4 Just before serving, top each meringue with 1 scant teaspoon of whipped topping and a strawberry.

Per serving: Kcalories 13 (From Fat 3); Fat 0g (Saturated 0g); Cholesterol 0mg; Sodium 6mg; Carbohydrate 2g (Dietary Fiber 1g); Protein 1g.

Enjoying a coffee break

Coffee is one of the most available beverages in society these days. You can't even take a stroll through your local grocery store or mall without being assaulted by the aromas of your local coffee roaster. And fortunately, most of them offer delicious decaffeinated versions of these aromatic beverages. Steam up a little nonfat milk to go with it, and you're ready to relax for a few minutes.

For a decadent but diabetic-friendly coffee break, make your own decaf, nonfat coffee drink (sweetened with sugar-free sweeteners, of course) and pair it with our delicious, crunchy biscotti.

Chocolate-Almond Biscotti

Prep time: 1 hr • **Cook time:** 45 min • **Yield:** 20 servings

Ingredients	Directions

Nonstick cooking spray

½ cup almonds, toasted and roughly chopped

½ cup all-purpose flour

⅓ cup whole-wheat flour

¼ cup unsweetened cocoa powder

2 teaspoons instant coffee crystals

½ teaspoon baking soda

⅛ teaspoon salt

½ cup Splenda for Baking

1 egg

1 egg white

1 teaspoon vanilla extract

1 teaspoon almond extract

1 Preheat the oven to 350 degrees. Line a large baking sheet with aluminum foil. Spray the foil with nonstick cooking spray.

2 In a food processor, combine ¼ cup of the almonds and the all-purpose flour, whole-wheat flour, cocoa powder, coffee crystals, baking soda, and salt. Process until the nuts are finely ground, approximately 2 minutes. Transfer the mixture to a large mixing bowl.

3 In the food processor, combine the Splenda, egg, egg white, vanilla extract, and almond extract. Mix until the mixture is slightly thickened, roughly 2 minutes. Add the egg mixture to the flour mixture in the mixing bowl. Stir in the remaining ¼ cup almonds.

4 Use half the batter to form a log (approximately 5 to 7 inches long) on one-half of the foil-lined baking sheet. Repeat with the remaining dough on other half of the baking sheet. Bake until firm, approximately 15 minutes. Cool approximately 10 minutes. Reduce the oven temperature to 300 degrees.

5 Place the logs on a cutting board. Using a serrated bread knife, cut each log into approximately 10 ½-inch diagonal slices. Return the slices to the baking sheets. Bake until the cut sides feel dry to the touch, approximately 20 minutes. Cool completely and store in an airtight container.

*Per serving (**1 biscotti**): Kcalories 60 (From Fat 15); Fat 2g (Saturated 0g); Cholesterol 11mg; Sodium 30mg; Carbohydrate 10g (Dietary Fiber 1g); Protein 2g.*

Part III
Eating Healthy Away from Home

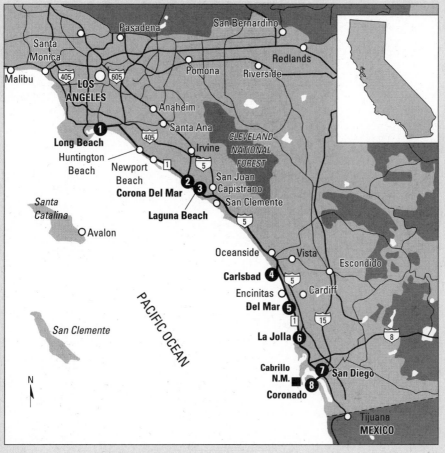

© John Wiley & Sons, Inc.

Understand the impact of exercise on diabetes in an article at www.dummies.com/extras/diabetescookbook.

In this part . . .

- ✔ Eat out without guilt.
- ✔ Enlist your host to help you eat right.
- ✔ Use nutritional information from fast food restaurants.
- ✔ Eat on the road.

Chapter 17

Making Eating Out a Nourishing Experience

*P*eople eat many of their meals in restaurants these days, so integrating restaurant eating into a nutritional plan is essential for a person with diabetes. The restaurant business is booming, and creative chefs have the same celebrity status as famous sports stars. And they deserve it. They use fresh ingredients to produce some of the most delicious and unique tastes imaginable. Unfortunately, nutrition isn't always uppermost in their minds. Our experience with the many chefs in this book proves that interest in good nutrition is increasing, but you're still on your own most of the time when selecting healthy foods. This chapter helps you ensure that your restaurant eating fits well into your nutritional plan.

Your situation may be much like the plight of the customer who called the waiter over and said, "Waiter, taste this soup." The waiter replied, "Is there something wrong with it?" "Never mind," said the customer, "just taste the soup." "But it smells and looks okay," said the waiter. "That's all right, just taste the soup," replied the customer. "But sir, there's no spoon," said the waiter. "Aha," said the customer. Or you may be like the diner who complains to the waiter, "Waiter, I can't find any steak in this steak pie." The waiter replies, "Well, there's no horse in the horseradish either." And if you find a fly in your soup, thank the waiter for the extra protein but ask him to serve it separately. The point is that you are ultimately responsible to ensure that you know what is in the food you order and make healthy choices.

Preparing for Restaurant Dining

If you live in (or are visiting) one of the cities that contains a restaurant we reference in this book (see Appendix A), the task of finding a restaurant that is appropriate for a person with diabetes is much easier for you. The chefs who have contributed to this book are health-conscious. They make an effort to keep the fat and the sugar low. But they have to respond to what they perceive to be their customers' needs. They think that one of the main "needs" is for a lot of food, so your portions will almost always be larger than necessary.

You have to evaluate the food you order by questioning your waitperson carefully. Even if the balance of energy sources is right, you will probably receive too much food and should take some home or leave some on your plate.

Because this book is limited to certain cities and restaurants, you may often find yourself having to choose a restaurant where you don't know the ingredients in the food or whether the menu items are healthy or not. How do you go about choosing a restaurant in this situation? Here are a few suggestions:

✔ No particular kind of food is better or worse than any other, with the exception of fast food (we discuss this issue in Chapter 18). You may think that vegetarian food is better than animal sources, but a dish of pasta in a creamy sauce is no better than a piece of fatty steak. Often, restaurants have several menu items that fit into your nutrition plan.

✔ Consider choosing a restaurant that you can walk to and from. The exercise you get will offset the extra calories you may consume.

✔ Many restaurants now publish their menus on the Internet. Before deciding to visit a particular restaurant, go to the establishment's website and make sure that it serves food you can eat.

✔ Don't go to the restaurant if the catch of the day is fish sticks.

✔ Call ahead and find out whether you can substitute items on the menu. Nonfranchise and non-fast-food restaurants are much more likely to let you substitute menu items. Fast-food restaurants are able to serve large numbers of people at lower prices by making the food entirely uniform. On the other hand, as Chapter 18 explains, this uniformity makes it easier to know the exact ingredients and methods of preparation. You need to ask only a few questions to know whether a restaurant will be accommodating. Ask whether the staff will

• Substitute skim milk for whole milk.

• Reduce the amount of butter and sugar in a dish.

• Serve gravies, salad dressings, and sauces on the side.

• Bake, broil, and poach instead of frying or sautéing.

✔ An older restaurant has the advantage of having experienced and well-trained waitstaff who know what the kitchen staff are willing to do for you, based on what has been done before.

✔ Find out whether the restaurant already has special meals or entrees for people with chronic diseases such as heart disease. They're much more likely to be health conscious in their cooking.

✔ When you choose a restaurant, consider what you've already eaten that day. For example, if you've already eaten your daily limit of carbohydrate, then the choice of a restaurant where pasta or rice is the major ingredient may not be a good one. People often choose a restaurant days in advance, so if you know ahead where you'll be dining, you can plan to modify your eating accordingly earlier in the day, especially if the restaurant specializes in foods you should eat in small quantities.

✔ Drink water or have a vegetable snack before you go to the restaurant so that hunger won't drive you to make bad choices.

✔ If you know that the restaurant serves huge portions of everything, don't go there unless you plan to share your meal or take part of your meal home.

Mrs. Wilson, who has type 2 diabetes, decided to go to a well-known delicatessen before she attended a musical play. She knew that they served huge portions, but she also knew that she could order a mini-version of many of the items. At the restaurant, she ordered a mini-Reuben sandwich, expecting to get half or less of the usual entree. What arrived was the entire Reuben sandwich without the usual potato salad and coleslaw. She couldn't take half of it home because she was going directly to the show. She knew that she'd feel bad leaving part of such a delicious sandwich, so she ended up eating most of it. Her blood glucose level later that night reflected the huge excess in calories that she had consumed.

You can see from the information in this section that you can do plenty, even before you reach the restaurant, to prepare for dining out. Your preparation may make the whole experience much more satisfying and less frustrating.

Starting the Meal

As you sit down to enjoy your meal, you can take many steps to make the experience of eating out the pleasure that it ought to be. A few simple considerations at this point allow you to enjoy the meal free of the concern that you are wrecking your nutritional program. Among the steps that you can take are the following:

✔ If you arrive early, avoid sitting in the bar with cocktails before you move to your table to eat your meal.

✔ Ask the hostess to seat you promptly so you don't have to wait and get too hungry or even hypoglycemic.

✔ Ask your waiter not to bring bread or to take it off the table if it is there already. That goes for chips and crackers as well.

✔ Ask for raw vegetables without a dip, what the restaurant menus call *crudités,* so you can munch on something before you order.

✔ Check your blood glucose before you order so you'll know how much carbohydrate is appropriate at that time.

✔ Wait to administer your short-acting insulin until you can be sure of the food delivery time.

Mr. Phillips, a 63-year-old man with type 2 diabetes, was trying to understand, with the help of his dietitian, why his blood glucose had risen to 386 mg/dl after a meal at a local Mexican restaurant. "I knew the portions were large, so I ordered a bean tortilla, and I didn't even eat the whole thing. I left half of it on my plate. I ate very little of the rice as well." The dietitian asked him if he had arrived early at the restaurant. "Oh yes, I forgot. I had to wait in the bar, and I had a virgin margarita." "That," said the dietitian, "explains your high blood glucose. The margarita is all carbohydrate."

Checking Out the Menu

The regular menu and the specials of the day or season are arranged to encourage you to order a big meal. One of the more interesting things that we learned as a result of working with the chefs whose recipes are found in this book, especially the European chefs now cooking in the United States, is the expectation of large portions on the part of U.S. restaurant-goers, compared to Europeans. The chefs were amazed at how much food they had to put on each plate to satisfy U.S. tastes. When you order meat, fish, or poultry, you often get at least twice as much as the recommended serving. Considering how frequently people eat out in the United States, it's no wonder the population is getting fatter.

Your strategy for ordering from the menu should include the following:

✔ Plan to leave some food or take home half your order, because the portions are always too large. You can also order a dish to share with another person.

✔ If you decide to have wine, order it by the glass. Diners almost always finish a bottle of wine, and unless eight of you share the bottle, you'll drink too much.

✔ Consider using an appetizer as your entree.

✔ Feel free to get a complete description, including portion size, of an appetizer or entree from the waitperson so that you aren't surprised when the food arrives. Pay particular attention to how the food is cooked — in fat or butter, for example.

✔ Consider a meal of soup and salad. This combination can be delicious, filling, low in calories, and low in carbohydrates.

✔ Order clear soups rather than cream soups.

✔ Ask for salad dressings and sauces on the side if possible. This way, you are in control of the amount you consume.

✔ You're probably wise to choose fish more often than meat, both to avoid fat and to take advantage of the cholesterol-lowering properties of fish. Remember, however, that fried fish can be as fat-laden as a steak.

✔ Let your server know that you need to eat soon. If your food will be delayed because the kitchen is slow or busy, insist that vegetable snacks be brought to the table.

The description of an entree usually offers clues that tell you whether it's a good choice for you. These words, in particular, indicate that the preparation keeps fat to a minimum:

✔ Baked

✔ Blackened

✔ Broiled

✔ Cooked in its own juice

✔ Grilled

✔ Poached

On the other hand, the following words point to a less desirable high-fat entree:

✔ Battered

✔ Buttered or in butter sauce

✔ Creamed or in cream sauce

✔ Deep-fried

✔ Escalloped

✔ Fried

✔ Golden brown

✔ In a plum sauce

✔ In cheese sauce

✔ Sautéed

✔ Sweet-and-sour

✔ With peanuts or cashews

Does it really matter if you order one kind of sauce versus another? Here are the calorie counts per tablespoon for various salad dressings. Remember that the energy in food is properly expressed in kilocalories, not calories, which are a thousand times smaller:

- ✔ **Blue cheese:** 82 kilocalories
- ✔ **Creamy Italian dressing:** 52 kilocalories
- ✔ **Lowfat French dressing:** 22 kilocalories
- ✔ **Red-wine vinegar:** 2 kilocalories

Planning at Each Meal and in Specific Kinds of Restaurants

You can make good choices at every meal, whether it's breakfast, lunch, or dinner. Every kind of food offers you the opportunity to select a lowfat, low-salt alternative. You just need to think about it and be aware of the possibilities. Helping you choose healthy meals is the purpose of this section.

Breakfast

The good choices at breakfast are fresh foods, which usually contain plenty of fiber. Fresh fruit is a good way to start the meal, followed by hot cereals such as oatmeal or Wheatena, or high-fiber cold cereals such as shredded wheat or bran cereals. Always add skim milk or 1 percent fat milk instead of whole milk. Enjoy egg whites but not yolks, or make an omelet with two whites for every yolk.

Less desirable choices are foods such as quiche, bacon, fried or hash brown potatoes, croissants, pastries, and doughnuts. And be careful of the high-calorie coffees. According to Starbucks's own website, a Strawberries and Crème Frappuccino Blended Crème-Whip has 570 kilocalories, including 130 kilocalories of fat.

Appetizers, salads, and soups

Raw and plain food beats those cooked and covered with butter or sour cream, and that rule applies to appetizers, salads, and soups, too. Raw carrots and celery can be enjoyed at any time and to almost any extent. Clear soups are always healthier. Salsa has become a popular accompaniment for crackers and chips instead of a high-fat dip. A delicious green salad is nutritious and filling.

By contrast, olives, nachos, and avocados have lots of fat. Nuts, chips, and cheese before dinner add lots of calories. Fried onion appetizers are currently very popular, and they're often dripping with fat. Watch out for the sour cream dips and the mayonnaise dips, since they, too, are full of fat.

Vegetarian food

As the population gets increasingly obese, there has been a trend to go to vegetarian restaurants. What is called vegetarian varies from no animal products at all, which is referred to as *vegan,* to eating eggs and/or dairy. Vegan diets can provide all the nutritional needs of a patient, but must be carefully planned to do so. Alternatively, vegan dieters can take supplements of calcium, iodine, vitamin B12, and vitamin D.

Lacto vegetarians eat dairy but not eggs while lacto-ovo vegetarians eat eggs and milk. Semi-vegetarians eat some fish and poultry as well.

Wherever you fit in the continuum of vegetarians, you should know that your choice is a good one. In general, vegetarians are lighter in weight than non-vegetarians. If you have diabetes, it is easier to control, and if you are at risk for diabetes, you are less likely to get it if you eat vegetarian. Vegetarian eating is also associated with less cancer, strokes, and heart attacks.

You still have to make good choices in the vegetarian restaurant. Stay away from the creamy, buttery foods and enjoy the lighter dishes made with grains like quinoa. Use beans and lentils to get your protein without the accompanying fat of meat.

Seafood

Most fish are relatively low in fat and can be a healthy choice. But even the best fish can compromise your nutrition plan when they're fried. Fish that stand out in the lowfat category are cod, bass, halibut, swordfish, and tuna in water. Most of the shellfish varieties are also lowfat. Stay away from herring, tuna in oil, and fried anything.

Chinese food

You can eat some great Chinese food and not have to worry about upsetting your diet plan. Any of the soups on the menu will be delicious and fill you up. Stick to vegetable dishes with small amounts of meat in them. Avoid fried dishes, whether they're meats, tofu, or rice and noodles. Steamed dishes are a much better choice. Potstickers, an appetizer often found on the menu, and sweet-and-sour pork will really throw off your calorie count and your fat intake. Stay away from the almond cookies that often follow Chinese meals.

French food

While the old style of preparing French food promotes a lot of cream and gravy, a new style, called the new cuisine, emphasizes the freshest ingredients, usually cooked in their own sauce. This style has revolutionized the French restaurants. Still, some French chefs cling to the old ways, and their food is not for you, unless you're prepared to share your meal.

Most desserts in French restaurants are high in carbohydrate. Limit yourself to a taste or, better yet, don't tempt yourself by ordering the cake or custard in the first place. See if the pastry chef has a fruit dish, like a poached pear, that is both delicious and good for you.

Indian food

Rice and pita bread are good carbohydrate choices, but avoid foods made with coconut milk because of its fat content. Meat, fish, and poultry cooked in the tandoori manner (baked in an oven) are fine, but Indian chefs like to fry many foods; keep those to a minimum. Curries are fine as long as they're not made with coconut milk. Avoid ghee, which is clarified butter. Fried appetizers like samosas and creamy dishes do not help your blood glucose. Chicken tikka and chapatti are fine — they're made with delicious spices (for taste) but little fat.

Italian food

Stick to tomato-based sauces and avoid the creamy, buttery, cheesy sauces. Minestrone soup is a hearty vegetable soup that is low in fat. Pasta, particularly whole-grain pasta, in general is fine as long as the sauce isn't fatty. The problem with the pasta, however, is that the quantity is almost always too great. Share it or take half home. Sausage, because of all the added fats, is a poor choice, whether served with pasta or placed on pizza. Pesto sauce can be made with little fat. If you love the taste of basil, as Dr. Rubin does, ask for a lowfat version of this classic sauce. Ask whether the kitchen staff will make garlic bread with roasted garlic alone, without the butter that often accompanies it. You'll be delighted with the delicious taste. Avoid Caesar salad and dishes made with a lot of cheese, such as cheese-filled ravioli.

Mexican food

Mexican food has become increasingly popular, but Mexican restaurants offer you many temptations to slip from your healthy eating plan. They often start with chips, nachos, and cheese. Tell your waiter to keep them off the table. Have salsa, not guacamole, as an appetizer. Stay away from anything refried; it means just what the word says. Avoid all dishes laden with cheese, as well as dishes heavy in sausage. Chicken with rice, grilled fish, and grilled chicken are excellent choices. Tortillas, burritos, and tostadas are delicious and good for you as long as you avoid the addition of a lot of cheese, sour cream, or guacamole. And keep in mind the importance of moderation. Mexican restaurants are known for large servings, so take some home.

Thai food

Other than the tendency to provide larger-than-needed portions, there is little that Thai restaurants do that is not good for the person with diabetes. The creative use of spices, emphasis on fish, and use of fresh vegetables make this cuisine a good choice for you. Just watch out for the hot spices.

Taking Pleasure in Your Food

If you've been conscientious in planning a delicious restaurant meal ahead of time, you deserve to really enjoy the food. But you need to continue thinking about healthy eating (and drinking) habits even as you sit down to the meal. All the great planning can come undone if you're careless at this point. Think about the following advice as you eat:

- ✔ If you have a glass of wine, consider the number of calories.

- ✔ Try using some behavior modification to prolong the meal and give your brain a chance to know that you've eaten: Eat slowly, chew each bite thoroughly, and put your fork down between each bite.

- ✔ Remember that the meal is a social occasion. Spend more time talking to your companions and less time concentrating on the food.

- ✔ Remove the skin if you're eating poultry, and allow the sauce to drip off the morsel of food on your fork if you're eating a dish cooked in a sauce.

- ✔ After you've carefully controlled the intake of food on your plate, don't add significant calories by tasting or finishing the food on your companion's plate.

Concluding with Dessert

For many people, the early parts of a meal are just a prelude to their favorite part, which is dessert. Most people have a sweet tooth, and dessert is often the way that they satisfy that need. The Italians don't call the part of the menu that features the desserts the *dulci* (which means "sweets") without reason. Dessert, in many restaurants, has become a showpiece. The pastry chef tries to show how sweet he or she can make the dessert while creating a culinary work of art. The term *decadent* is often used in describing the richness of these desserts.

Does this mean that you can't have any dessert at all? No. Making a wise choice simply requires a certain amount of awareness on your part. You need to ask yourself the question, "Is the taste of this dessert worth the potential damage it will do to my blood glucose and calorie intake?" If you can answer this question with a "yes," then have the dessert, but check your blood glucose and adjust your medications as needed after eating it. Then return to your nutritional plan without spending a lot of time regretting your lapse. You might even do a little extra exercise to counteract the calories.

On the other hand, if you want to answer the question with a "no," ask yourself these questions to help you avoid temptation:

✔ Do you really need or want the dessert?

✔ Will you remember it ten minutes later when you're at the theater?

✔ Could you share the dessert or just taste it?

✔ Is a fruit dessert available that you could enjoy instead?

To help you avoid that high-calorie dessert even further, think in terms of the number of minutes of active aerobic exercise you must do to account for the calories you consume in a dessert. If your exercise is walking, double these times. Here are some examples:

✔ Boston cream pie: 32 minutes

✔ Brownie: 32 minutes

✔ Apple pie: 34 minutes

✔ Hot fudge sundae: 38 minutes

✔ Cheesecake: 40 minutes

✔ Ice cream cone: 44 minutes

✔ Strawberry milkshake: 47 minutes

You may conclude that dessert is worth your time, but we'll leave that decision up to you.

Chapter 18

Fast Food on Your Itinerary

. . . .

In This Chapter

▶ Getting a feel for fast-food options

▶ Touring the east coast of Florida

▶ Heading down the western side of Georgia

▶ Checking out Baltimore and Annapolis

▶ Finding there's no place like Kansas

▶ Traveling from Los Angeles to San Diego along the Pacific Coast Highway

. . . .

*W*ould you like to take a ride with Dr. Rubin and Cait? Here's your chance. You're invited to travel with them on the highways and byways of some of the most scenic areas of the country with the best destinations. You will stop along the way at some of the best-known fast-food restaurants. Luckily, you are with Cait, who knows the contents of all the foods in these restaurants, and Dr. Rubin, who is there to make sure that you enjoy yourself while staying on your eating program. If you want to get the details on these trips, you'll need to check out travel guidebooks on the areas that interest you. We give you just the bare essentials here.

We selected these specific restaurants because they're usually the most common examples of a particular class of fast-food restaurants. In no way do we mean to recommend them above others in their class.

In this chapter, we hit the high spots, the most commonly visited fast-food places. Keep in mind that one chapter isn't enough space to cover the hundreds of different fast-food franchises all over the country. In general, a burger in McDonald's looks like a burger at Burger King, but there are major variations.

A number of things about fast food should be clear from our driving tours of the United States:

✔ There are very few choices on fast-food menus that are healthy for you as a diabetic.

✔ Most entrees have too much fat and too much salt.

✔ You usually have to check the salads with some protein such as chicken or shrimp to find something you can eat.

✔ Salads should be accompanied by lowfat dressing.

✔ An occasional dessert that you share is okay. Otherwise, stick to sorbet.

✔ Bring your own fruit for a better choice.

✔ If you go where you have no nutritional information, sharing the food reduces the calories, fat, and salt.

Touring the Fast-Food Landscape

Is it even important to discuss fast-food restaurants? McDonald's claims that it serves 6 million customers every day in the United States. That's almost one in ten of all Americans. It has over 34,000 restaurants, compared with over 11,000 for Burger King; 5,900 for Wendy's; and 3,600 for Arby's. You bet they have a huge impact on eating in America.

People used to say that at fast-food restaurants you could get more nourishment from biting your lip than eating the food. This is definitely no longer the case. Because everyone is conscious of good nutrition these days, you can now find something healthful to eat in any fast-food restaurant.

Watch for a few key words that warn you not to order a particular item in these restaurants. If the food is called a double, big, jumbo, monster, or the ultimate, stay away from that selection. Also avoid any menu item with bacon or sausage.

The reason these establishments are called fast-food restaurants is that they have food preparation, ordering, and serving down to the least amount of time possible. Because we're in a hurry on our trips in this chapter and don't want to stop for a long time, there's nothing wrong with enjoying that convenience, but we want to make sure that the food is right for you.

Of course, some of these places aren't meant to rush into and out of. They are sit-down places, but the food is standardized and is prepared pretty fast, so the result is about the same. This chapter discusses those kinds of restaurants, too.

One advantage of franchise restaurants is that a hamburger in a Denny's in California is almost exactly the same as a hamburger in a Denny's in New Mexico or Oregon. You know exactly what you're getting, which makes the meal easier to fit into your diet. On the other hand, the quick serving and eating often doesn't allow your brain enough time to recognize that your body has eaten enough calories, and you may be tempted to order more food. Don't.

A study published in *The Lancet* in December 2004 that followed 3,000 people over 15 years showed that those who ate regularly at fast-food restaurants gained 10 pounds more than those who did not and were much more likely to develop diabetes. They did not have Cait and Dr. Rubin along to help them as you do. Cait has selected the restaurants in advance to save you the trouble of choosing them along the way.

In Chapter 2, we introduce you to trans fats, the absolutely worst kind of fat, because it not only raises bad cholesterol but lowers good cholesterol. These fats are also called hydrogenated or partially hydrogenated oils. Since 2006, food labels have had to list the amount of trans fats, and the better fast-food places are trying to eliminate them from their cooking. They're still present in large amounts, however, especially in foods like french-fried potatoes, batter-dipped fried onions, fried mozzarella sticks, and buffalo wings. The best way to avoid trans fats is to order food that is low in all fats. The fast-food restaurants that have *no* trans fats in their foods include:

- ✔ In-N-Out Burger
- ✔ Subway
- ✔ McDonald's
- ✔ KFC
- ✔ Pizza Hut
- ✔ Popeyes
- ✔ Little Caesars
- ✔ Papa Johns

The fast-food restaurants that are the worst offenders with the most items with trans fats are:

- ✔ Jack in the Box
- ✔ Taco Bell
- ✔ White Castle
- ✔ A & W
- ✔ Dairy Queen

On the trips we're going to take in this chapter, we're going to avoid the heavy offenders and emphasize the zero users.

No one should say that a person with diabetes can't go to a fast-food restaurant and remain on his or her nutritional plan. But these places do offer many seductive and unhealthy choices. You need to plan in advance what you're going to choose. You can't go wrong if you stick to the selections that we talk about in this chapter.

Don't make a habit of eating at fast-food restaurants. Although they may be a convenience on the road, they aren't good for you long term. Here are some reasons:

- ✔ Where fast-food consumption is high, so is obesity and the incidence of diabetes.

- ✔ Analysis of children's meals at 22 fast-food restaurants revealed that 99 percent were of poor nutritional quality based on nutrition recommendations in the Dietary Guidelines for Americans.

- ✔ Despite recommendations that the kilocalorie counts of fast foods should be reduced, they remain unchanged after a decade. So, leave some on your tray.

If you want to be sure of the nutritional *content* of various fast foods, refer to your favorite search engine on the Internet and enter the name of a specific franchise. All the details are there. Unfortunately, some sites leave out one or another of the nutrients. What you find in this chapter is what each chain offers.

Driving along the Atlantic Coast of Florida

This trip should be planned from November to May to avoid the heat of summer. It's a total distance of 130 miles (see Figure 18-1).

We begin in Boca Raton, which was developed by Addison Mizner in the 1920s. It and the rest of the tour are located on the A1A highway along the east coast of Florida. At the Town Hall Museum, we can get a good idea of how Boca was developed. There is a good collection of 20th-century artists at the Boca Raton Museum of Art. Because we're interested in the environment, we may want to take a look at the Gumbo Limbo Nature Center, dedicated to preservation of the turtles of the coast.

We continue on the A1A for 30 miles to Palm Beach, the richest community on this tour. We don't want to miss the Henry Morrison Flagler Museum, a mansion built by the cofounder of Standard Oil. The Breakers is the magnificent resort located in Palm Beach on 140 beachfront acres. It was also founded by Henry Flagler and has all the amenities of the best resorts. We plan to stop in for a cup of tea at least.

You won't find many fast-food restaurants around here — they don't encourage them. So, we get back on the A1A and head a little farther north to Riviera Beach where we find a McDonald's. Cait says if we want to stay close to our Mediterranean diet, we have to avoid McDonald's burgers. She spots the Premium Southwest Salad with Grilled Chicken (avoid the fat-filled Crispy Chicken), which has a total of 290 kilocalories, 70 of which are fat but just 2.5 g of saturated fat and no trans fat. It has 70 mg of cholesterol and 28 g of carbohydrates. Its one downside is its 650 mg of sodium. We can enjoy some apple slices with our salad.

We stay overnight in the area and spend the next day in West Palm Beach, not surprisingly just to the west of Palm Beach. Here we visit the Ann Norton Sculpture Garden and the Norton Museum of Art. Stroll down Clematis Street for the shops and the nightlife. Then we get back on the A1A and head north to Jupiter, where the islands disappear and A1A is on the mainland. We visit a pioneer home from the 19th century called DuBois House and the Florida History Center and Museum and end up at the Jupiter Inlet Lighthouse.

In Jupiter, we find Papa John's. The best choice here is probably the medium Garden Fresh Original Crust Pizza with 200 kilocalories, 7 g of fat, 3 g of saturated fat, 15 mg of cholesterol, 27 g of carbohydrates, and 500 mg of sodium. Stick to water for your beverage or have a diet soda — just avoid a lot of added sugar. Papa John's offers nothing that we should eat for dessert. We're prepared for this and travel with fresh fruit. We won't find it in fast-food restaurants. A banana would be a good finish to our meal.

We stay overnight and head farther up the A1A to Hutchinson Island and Jensen Beach, another center for sea turtles. We go a few miles farther up to Fort Pierce, where we find the Heathcote Botanical Gardens and the National Navy UDT-SEAL Museum, where 3,000 navy frogmen trained during World War II. We end our tour in Vero Beach. The Environmental Learning Center is a great place to learn about the fish and the flora of the area. And we end our eating at the Outback Steakhouse. We won't be having steak; instead, we'll go with the salmon. It has 480 kilocalories, 29 g of fat, 6 g of saturated fat, 65 mg of cholesterol, 14 g of carbohydrate, and 450 mg of sodium. This meal is the best we've had yet.

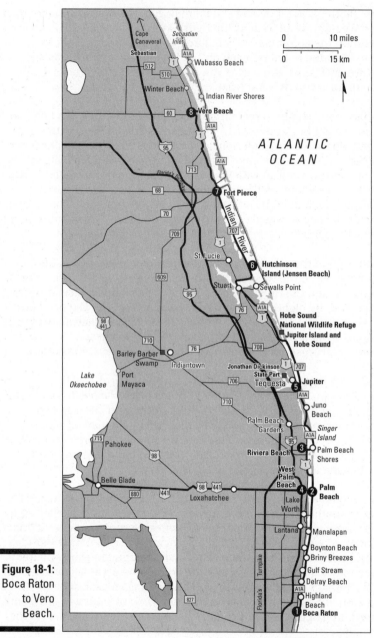

Figure 18-1:
Boca Raton
to Vero
Beach.

Georgia, Down the West Side of the State

We want to take this trip (see Figure 18-2) in the spring or fall because we don't love heat and humidity. We start in the northwest corner of the state in Rossville, where a Cherokee Indian named John Ross fought for years (unsuccessfully) to keep his tribe from being moved to Oklahoma. His wife died on the march. We visit his house, and then go south on U.S. 27 (also known as State Route 1) to the oldest military park in the nation, the Chickamauga and Chattanooga National Military Park, where we learn about one of the bloodiest battles of the Civil War.

We continue south and stop at Paradise Gardens, where we view the folk-art paintings of Harold Finster. U.S. 27 passes through the huge Chattahoochee National Forest and continues on to Rome, built on seven hills (like that somewhat larger city in Italy). Right along this road in Rome, we stop at Arby's. Although Arby's is known for roast beef, we're avoiding red meat. Instead, we have the Chopped Farmhouse Salad with Roast Turkey and dress it with oil and vinegar (because even the Light Italian Dressing, though low in calories and fat, has way too much sodium). The salad has 230 kilocalories (120 from fat). There are 13 g of fat, 7 g of saturated fat, 60 mg of cholesterol, and a whopping 780 mg of sodium. Somebody needs to control the salt shaker! (The Dietary Guidelines for Americans recommends no more salt than 2,300 mg of sodium per day.) Arby's offers some apple slices like McDonald's, so we take advantage of that.

Staying overnight in Rome, we continue south the next morning to Carrollton, named after John Carroll, who signed the Declaration of Independence. Still farther south is LaGrange, where we can visit Bellevue, the home of Benjamin Harvey Hill, a prominent U.S. and Confederate politician before the Civil War. We check out the Chattahoochee Art Museum, which was converted from a jail. We will see 20th-century American art.

Twenty miles south of LaGrange is Pine Mountain, where the lovely Callaway Gardens will please our senses. Within the gardens is the Cecil B. Day Butterfly Center. Next is Columbus, the home of the National Infantry Museum and the Port Columbus Civil War Naval Center. In Columbus, we stop at Houlihan's. There are only 84 of them in the country, but the menu is similar to the larger chains. Cait suggests the Fish Tacos Combo. At 438 kilocalories, it has 20 g of fat, 4 g of saturated fat, 45 g of carbohydrate, and 844 mg of sodium. You'll want to dig in to your fruit basket for a nice pear or an apple.

Columbus is another good place to spend the night. Then we head south to Westville, which is a reconstructed village featuring rural life in Georgia during the 19th century. A little farther south and we're in Florida. We've traveled about 360 miles.

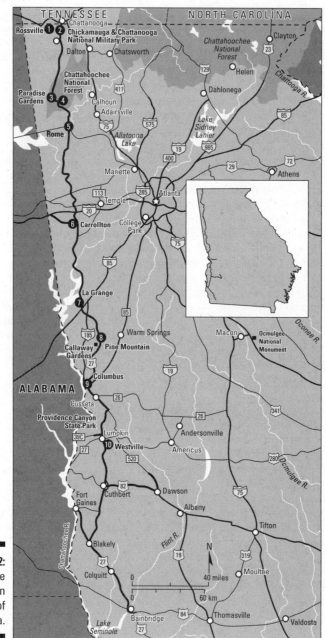

Figure 18-2:
Down the
western
side of
Georgia.

Maryland: Baltimore and Annapolis

This trip (see Figure 18-3) is short (73 miles) but very historic. It's best made in the spring or fall.

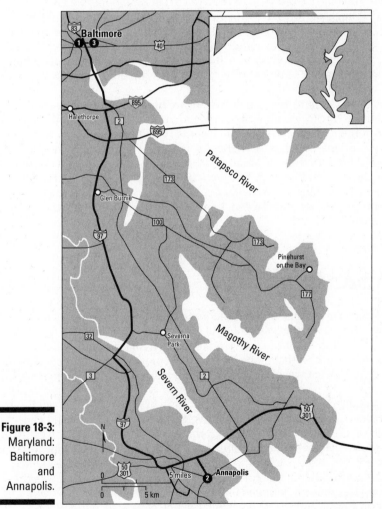

Figure 18-3:
Maryland:
Baltimore
and
Annapolis.

© John Wiley & Sons, Inc.

We start at Baltimore's Inner Harbor. We haven't done much shopping so far, so Harborplace would be a good place to get the T-shirts we want for our kids. We go to the National Aquarium and the National Science Center for some brain stimulation. We should also visit the American Visionary Art Museum before leaving Inner Harbor.

To get to Annapolis, we take I-95 to I-695 to I-97. In Annapolis, we visit P.F. Chang's. Cait suggests we start with a cup of wonton soup at only 50 kilocalories, 1 g of fat, 8 g of carbohydrates, and 720 mg of sodium. The spicy ahi tuna roll should be enjoyable and do little damage with its 280 kilocalories, 3 g of fat, and 45 g of carbohydrates. It has an unfortunate 930 mg of sodium, though, so we won't be eating at other P.F. Chang's on our driving adventures.

Annapolis offers a ton to see and do. There are historic houses like the Maryland State House, which was completed in 1780; the Hammond-Harwood House, 90 percent of which is original from 1774; and the London Town House and Gardens, which is an archeological site. The United States Naval Academy offers tours from the visitor center, which has exhibits of the life of the midshipmen and women. We have to show a photo ID to get in. Within the Academy is the Museum & Gallery of Ships. In addition, we want to see the William Paca House and Garden, honoring a signer of the Declaration of Independence.

Along the Santa Fe Trail

After the short trip we took from Baltimore to Annapolis, we're ready for a much longer ride along the Santa Fe Trail (see Figure 18-4). This 427-mile tour follows U.S. 56 southwest from Edgerton to Elkhart, Kansas, cutting Kansas in half. It was the direction that many thousands of pioneers took from east of the Missouri River to what was then the Mexican territories starting in the 1820s.

We begin in Edgerton and stop at Baldwin City, where we visit the Ivan Boyd Prairie Preserve. We learn about the native grasses of the prairie and can see actual wagon ruts from the long-ago wagon trains. We continue west to Council Grove, filled with historic sites from the trail. We see the Kaw Mission State Historic Site and learn about the Kaw Indians. We visit the Post Office Oak and Museum, where pioneers left messages in an oak tree that was the post office. The museum contains many artifacts from the time. The Old Calaboose is a replica of the original jail. Council Grove is a good place to spend the night but there are no fast-food restaurants, so we can go to Hays House 1857 Restaurant and Tavern, the oldest continuously operating restaurant west of the Mississippi. It's not a fast-food place and there is no nutrition information, but you can't go wrong if you *share* the catfish on the menu. Have a glass of Barefoot Pinot Grigio and *share* a piece of the cranberry-strawberry pie for a special treat.

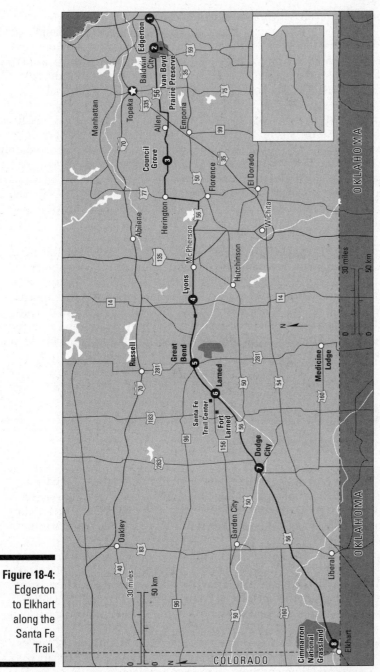

Figure 18-4:
Edgerton
to Elkhart
along the
Santa Fe
Trail.

© *John Wiley & Sons, Inc.*

We continue west on 56 to Lyons, where the Coronado Quivira Museum shows us how people lived on the trail. We head down to the city of Great Bend, where we learn much more about the Santa Fe Trail at the Barton County Historical Society Museum and Village. Next we reach Larned, 2 miles from the Santa Fe Trail Center, a research museum for the trail. We also visit the Fort Larned National Historic Site. Fort Larned was the guardian of the trail.

About 60 miles farther is Dodge City, the "wickedest city of the west." In the late 19th century, there was no local law enforcement. Buffalo hunters, railroad workers, drifters, and soldiers fought and killed one another. Fortunately, that is no longer the case, and there is a KFC in town, where we can have a meal. We aren't having the fried chicken — too much fat — but KFC also offers grilled chicken. A drumstick and a breast total 310 kilocalories (95 from fat), 11 g of fat, 3 g of saturated fat, 195 mg of cholesterol, and 1,020 mg of sodium. We stay in Dodge City overnight.

Two hours west of Dodge City, U.S. 56 and the Santa Fe Trail leave Kansas at Elkhart. The Cimarron National Grassland, the largest area of public land in Kansas, with over 108,000 acres, provides self-guided tours. There is a 30-mile auto tour. The Dust Bowl of the 1930s severely affected this area after wheat farmers dug up the prairie and planted their wheat. Years of drought followed. The federal government stepped in, bought the land, and restored the prairie, creating the Cimarron National Grassland. We do some hiking and camping while we're here.

Southern California along the Pacific Coast Highway

California is our home state, although we both live in Northern California. We've both traveled in California many times, but it never gets old. We're taking a 140-mile trip (see Figure 18-5) over two days with views, views, and views of the Pacific Ocean. The weather is fine all year long, but in winter the crowds are smaller.

We leave Los Angeles on I-405 south heading for Long Beach. We could stop right here for a week, but we take in just a few of the many sites. There is the Aquarium of the Pacific, the Museum of Latin American Art, and the Queen Mary Seaport, where the ship has been turned into a hotel and living museum.

At Long Beach, we begin on Route 1, the Pacific Coast Highway. In 22 miles, we're at Corona del Mar, one of the numerous beach towns we're visiting. We go for a swim and then continue on to Laguna Beach, 7 miles south. This town is a mixture of hippy, gay culture and rich, conservative folks. It's full of art galleries and antique shops. Crystal Cove State Park has hiking and biking, but the best feature is the 1,000-acre scuba park. We didn't bring our scuba gear, but we do a little snorkeling.

Route 1 ends at San Clemente, where former president Richard Nixon had his "Western White House," but he sold the property and lived elsewhere before he died. San Clemente is famous as a great site for surfing. We have to take I-5 to get to our next destination, Carlsbad, where we stay overnight.

There is a TGI Friday's in Carlsbad. Cait suggests we try it. TGI Friday's began in New York City as a singles bar, but today it has over 600 restaurants in the United States, serving pretty good food. It has an extensive menu, but when we check the nutritional information, most entrees have a lot of fat and/or salt. One exception is the Lunch Grilled Chicken Cobb Salad, to which we add the Low-Fat Balsamic Vinaigrette dressing. The kilocalorie count is 460, with 28 g of fat, 8 g of saturated fat, 20 g of carbohydrates, and 1,030 mg of sodium. We have the orange sherbet for an additional 130 kilocalories with 37 mg of carbohydrate.

Leaving Carlsbad, we go further south to Del Mar, "the toast of the coast." It has a racetrack that we won't visit and some lovely beaches. Ten miles more and we're in La Jolla, which is actually a part of San Diego. It has some of the best scuba diving, snorkeling, and surfing on this trip. It also has a Museum of Contemporary Art with great art and a great setting.

Finally, we reach San Diego with lots to see and do. Across the San Diego–Coronado Bay Bridge is the isthmus of Coronado with its Hotel Del Coronado, where the funniest movie ever made, *Some Like It Hot,* starring Marilyn Monroe, Tony Curtis, and Jack Lemmon, was made. Back in San Diego, we go through Balboa Park with its zoo, performances, and picnic areas. The Cabrillo National Monument recalls the site of the first European visitor to San Diego, Juan Rodriguez Cabrillo. It has 144 acres with plenty of hiking and great views. The Gaslamp Quarter near the harbor is filled with shops and restaurants. The Maritime Museum is also on our agenda; it has six restored ships and lots of history of the seaport. The San Diego Museum of Art has a great collection of Spanish and renaissance paintings and over 100 works by Toulouse-Lautrec.

Our final meal on this trip is at McCormick and Schmick's Seafood and Steaks. Although it has only 68 locations, it's a personal favorite of Dr. Rubin and a delicious way to end this travel by the sea. The restaurant does not offer specific nutritional information, but we're going to share the food, so we should be okay. The Grilled Pacific Swordfish stands out with a glass of Chardonnay to go with it. Seasonal sorbet for dessert shouldn't do too much damage to our eating program.

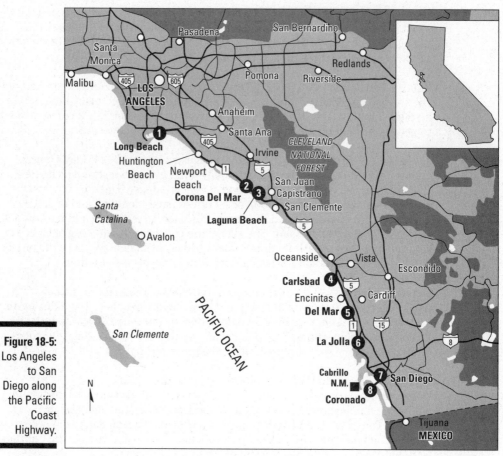

Figure 18-5:
Los Angeles
to San
Diego along
the Pacific
Coast
Highway.

Part IV
The Part of Tens

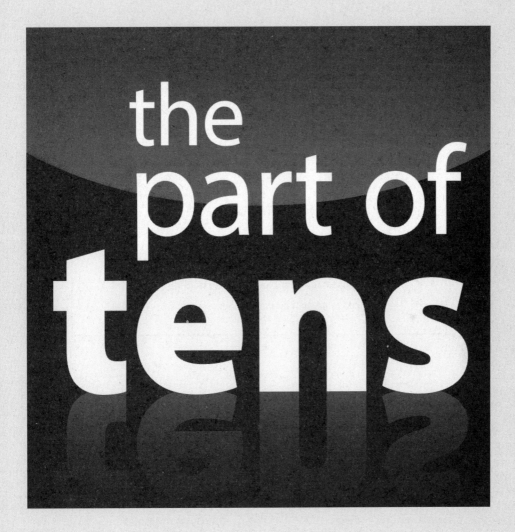

Find ten myths about diabetes in a free article at www.dummies.com/extras/diabetescookbook.

In this part . . .

- ✔ Make simple changes that pack a powerful punch.
- ✔ Find out how to switch to a Mediterranean diet.
- ✔ See what helps keep your blood glucose normal.
- ✔ Get your kids to enjoy their vegetables.

Chapter 19

Ten (Or So) Simple Steps to Change Your Eating Habits

*F*ollowing a nutritional plan sometimes seems so complicated. But really, if you follow the few simple rules outlined in this chapter, you can make the process much easier. This chapter provides you with ten (or so) simple things you can do today. None of them cost anything other than time. Doing them one at a time makes a big difference in your calorie and fat intake. Adding one after another makes the results huge. Your weight, blood pressure, and blood glucose all fall. Who could ask for anything more?

Enjoying a Good Breakfast

People often think that the path to weight loss is to skip meals, and breakfast is often the first to go. However, the "successful losers" in the National Weight Loss Registry would disagree: 78 percent of them eat a good breakfast and only 4 percent skip breakfast. Eating a healthy breakfast prevents much greater eating later in the day.

So, what's is a healthy breakfast? An easy option is whole-grain cereal with lowfat milk, and a piece of fruit. Some other suggestions include steel-cut oats with hemp protein powder, flaxseed, walnuts and fruit, or eggs with whole wheat toast and fruit. Avoid heavy breakfasts like pancakes, French toast, or waffles with sausage.

Still not convinced breakfast is for you? People who eat breakfast:

- ✔ Are better able to concentrate at work or in school
- ✔ Are stronger and can last longer doing physical activity
- ✔ Tend to eat a more nutritionally complete diet overall
- ✔ Have an easier time controlling their weight
- ✔ Have lower cholesterol
- ✔ Tend not to binge
- ✔ Tend to have a better mood

Limiting Quantities and Making Substitutions

In the typical Western diet, many foods are high in sugar, fat, salt, and calories, but low in nutrition. We're thinking here of alcohol, cakes, candies, chocolate, cookies, doughnuts, energy drinks, french fries, fruit-flavored drinks, granola bars (yes, even supposedly "healthy" granola bars), ice cream and other frozen desserts, muffins, nachos, pastries, potato chips, soft drinks, sports drinks, and more.

If you want to lose weight and/or improve your health, you have to severely limit or avoid these foods altogether. "What?", you say, "Impossible!" But what if we guaranteed you would live an additional three to five years. Well, we can't do that — there are no guarantees in life. But we can promise that you'll lose weight and feel better than you do now.

You can substitute a healthier food for just about any not-so-healthy food. Here are some examples:

Instead of . . .	Try . . .
Cakes or pastries	Fruit with yogurt or a baked apple
Chocolate, candies, cookies, granola, or potato chips	Popcorn with herbs
Doughnuts or muffins	High-fiber, whole-grain muffins
French fries	Potato strips baked with a little olive oil
Fruit-flavored drinks and soft drinks	Carbonated water with lemon or lime
Ice cream	Frozen lowfat yogurt
Nachos	Lowfat cheese melted on whole-grain chips
Energy drinks, sports drinks	Water with lemon or lime

Eating Every Meal

When you miss meals, you become hungry. If you have type 1 diabetes, you can't safely miss meals, especially if you give yourself regular or lispro insulin. Instead of letting yourself become hungry, eat your meals at regular times so that you don't overcompensate at the next meal (or at a snack shortly after the meal you missed) when you're suffering from low blood glucose. Many people overtreat low blood glucose by eating too many sugar calories, resulting in high blood glucose later on.

You should not miss meals as a weight-loss method, particularly if you take a drug that lowers blood glucose into hypoglycemic levels. A pregnant woman with diabetes especially should not miss meals. She must make up for the fact that her baby extracts large amounts of glucose from her blood. Both mother and growing fetus are adversely affected if the mother's body must turn to stored fat for energy.

Eating smaller meals and having snacks in between is probably the best way to eat because doing so raises blood glucose the least, provides a constant source of energy, and allows control of the blood glucose using the least amount of external or internal insulin.

The fact is, following your complete nutritional plan in fewer than three meals is extremely difficult.

Setting Specific Goals

If you planned to climb Mt. Everest, your itinerary would not read, "Arrive at the base, arrive at the top." In just the same way, the goals you set for losing weight and switching to the Mediterranean diet need to be achievable and very specific. For example, don't just set a goal to "Lose 40 pounds." You may be able to do it, eventually, but it's much more likely that you'll lose 5 pounds, and that should be your initial goal. After you've done that, you can plan to lose another 5 pounds, and so forth.

Goals should be very specific. For example, "I will eat fruit rather than cake for dessert" is a much better goal than "I will stop eating cake."

Choose goals that you have real control over. You're much more likely to succeed in reducing your fat intake than lowering your cholesterol, although reducing your fat intake may cause your cholesterol to go down. It's also helpful to choose goals you can easily measure, like your weight and the number of steps you walk each day.

Your goals should be forgiving. Don't beat yourself up if you don't succeed the first time around.

Here are some specific goals to get you started:

- ✔ I will chew my food thoroughly to reduce the pace of eating.
- ✔ I will leave some food on my plate at each meal.
- ✔ I will reduce my portions by one-third.
- ✔ I will eliminate second servings.
- ✔ I will make healthy substitutions.
- ✔ I will wear a pedometer and increase my daily steps by 100 until I reach 10,000 steps at least five days a week.
- ✔ I will give myself specific rewards for achieving my goals, but those rewards will never be food.
- ✔ I will use yoga, meditation, or some other technique to manage the stress that leads to overeating.

Drinking Water throughout the Day

Seventy percent of your body is water, and all your many organs and cells require water to function properly. Most people, especially older people, don't get enough water. Older people often have the additional disadvantage of losing their ability to sense when they're thirsty. The consequences may include weakness and fatigue, not to mention constipation.

Water can replace all the sodas and juice drinks that add unwanted calories to your day. You soon lose your taste for those drinks and discover that you don't need (or miss) the aftertaste of soda and juice that you took for granted. Those drinks also raise the blood glucose very rapidly and are often used to treat low blood glucose.

One of our patients admitted to drinking 10 to 12 cans of cola drinks daily. He had a high blood glucose that returned to normal when he broke his cola habit.

Make drinking water a part of your daily habits. Drink some when you brush your teeth. Drink more with meals and snacks. Many people don't want to drink much water close to bedtime because if they do, they'll have to get up during the night to go to the bathroom — all the more reason to make sure you get your daily water ration.

Reinforcing Your Behavior Change

One of the most supportive ways to change your behavior is with reinforcement. Reinforcement may be intrinsic (a pleasurable state of mind like happiness or satisfaction) or extrinsic (a new dress or money, for example). You need to figure out which reinforcements work best for you. Here are some key intrinsic motivators:

- ✔ **Acceptance:** You want to be accepted by your friends and society.
- ✔ **Curiosity:** You want to know the things that make you healthy.
- ✔ **Independence:** You want to believe that you can succeed on your own.
- ✔ **Power:** You want to feel that you have control over your own body.
- ✔ **Social contact:** You want to feel good enough about yourself to interact with others.
- ✔ **Social status:** You want to feel important in your society.

Any or all of these intrinsic motivators may be the force that gets you to follow a dietary program and do the necessary exercise. On the other hand, you may need tangible evidence of your success as well. Some of the strongest extrinsic motivators include the following:

- ✔ Money
- ✔ Gifts to yourself
- ✔ Activities that you enjoy

Obviously, food can't be an extrinsic motivator unless and until you realize that fruits or vegetables are the things that should give you the most pleasure and not the desserts you may have enjoyed in the past.

Removing the Attached Fat

Many foods, such as sausage and luncheon meats, contain so much fat that lowering their fat content isn't possible. You should mostly avoid these foods. But other protein sources, such as chicken, steak, roast beef, and pork, have large amounts of visible fat attached to them, so you can remove this fat before you prepare the food. In the case of poultry, removing the skin removes most of the fat. Selecting white meat rather than dark further reduces the fat in poultry.

As fat cooks on a grill, it often flames, which causes the meat to burn. Removing the fat before you cook it makes the cooking process safer (because the burning fat won't spray around), and the resulting meat is much lower in calories.

Leaving Out the Salt

For reasons that are unclear to us, most Americans like a lot of salt in their food. Consequently, these people taste mostly salt and not much of the food. Try getting rid of the salt in your recipes. You can always add it later if you miss the flavor that salt adds. At first, you may think that the food tastes bland. Then you'll begin to discover the subtle tastes that were in the food all along but were overpowered by the salt.

Why do we emphasize cutting salt levels? We know that salt raises blood pressure. Recent studies, particularly the United Kingdom Prospective Diabetes Study, which was a major breakthrough published in 1998, have shown that you can slow or prevent diabetic complications by reducing blood pressure.

You can try the approach of slowly removing salt from the recipe. If it calls for a teaspoon of salt, add only ¾ teaspoon. You won't notice the difference. Next time, try ½ teaspoon. And so on. In the recipes in this book, we have tried to use less salt wherever possible, with the permission of the chefs who created the recipes. Most chefs have been very open to eliminating salt. They use herbs, spices, and other flavors to replace salt.

Tracking Food with a Diary

Try this little diversion: For the next two days, write down everything you eat and drink. Before you go to bed on the evening of the second day, take a separate piece of paper and try to reconstruct what you've eaten for the past two days without looking at your original list. Then compare the two lists. The differences in the lists will startle you. The point of this exercise is to show you that you're doing a lot of mindless eating. Trying to follow a nutritional plan from memory doesn't work.

A food diary not only shows you what you're eating all the time but also makes it easy to select items to reduce in portion size or eliminate altogether. When you go to your doctor, the fact that your diary lists birdseed for every meal helps confirm your statement that you eat like a bird.

To really have an effect, a food diary must be complete. The more complete your diary, the more likely it will help you and any caregiver to understand when you succeed and when you don't. Here's the information that's most important in your food diary:

- All the foods and beverages you consumed during the day and night

- The amount in ounces, grams, or portions of each food

- How hungry you were when you ate the food (assign a number from 1, meaning stuffed, to 5, meaning extremely hungry)

- The time of day when you ate

- How you felt emotionally when you ate the food

- Your exercise for the day

- Your strategies for the following day

After you have all this information written down, you can begin to use the motivators described earlier in this chapter to reinforce your helpful eating and exercise behaviors. With this level of detail, you can calculate exactly how much you're eating and cut back if necessary. Finally, you can figure out if emotion plays a role (hint: it usually does).

Cooking by the B's

The best methods of cooking all begin with a *b:*

- **Braising:** Browning the ingredient first on top of the stove and then slowly cooking it partially covered with a small quantity of liquid like water or broth. The cooking liquid can be used to form a flavorful sauce.

- **Broiling and barbecuing:** Exposing the food to direct heat. When you broil, you place the food on a broiler rack below a heating element or flame. When you barbecue, you place the food on a grill above charcoals or a flame. Both techniques result in the fat dripping away.

- **Boiling:** Cooking food in boiling water. Boiling results in significant loss of fat as it melts away into the water.

These methods of preparation don't add fat and often remove a lot of the fat within the food. Broiling a hamburger, for example, often eliminates as much fat from a moderate-fat hamburger as buying a reduced-fat hamburger to begin with. Frying, sautéing, and other methods that depend on butter or fat add exactly the things that you want to remove.

It is possible to sauté food without using fat if you have a good nonstick pan. Then the fat in the food provides the "grease" to keep the food from sticking.

If you must use fat, use a cooking spray that reduces the amount of added fat.

Chapter 20

Ten Simple Steps to Adopting a Mediterranean Diet

. . . .

In This Chapter

▶ Giving up salt

▶ Switching to whole grains

▶ Substituting fish and poultry for meat

▶ Using olive oil in place of butter

▶ Enjoying vegetables throughout the day

▶ Switching to fruits instead of cakes

. . . .

*Y*ou may think that giving up the diet you've followed all your life in favor of the Mediterranean diet requires a major upheaval in your lifestyle. The process may not be simple, but we guarantee you aren't giving up good taste. We know you'll enjoy the diet — and your blood glucose, blood pressure, cholesterol, and weight will all take a turn for the better. In this chapter, you find ten ways to go from your current diet to the Mediterranean diet.

Giving Up Salt in Favor of Herbs and Spices

Most people eat too much salt. Just reducing the salt in your diet will help to bring down your blood pressure, but you may complain about the loss of flavor. The good news is, you can add herbs and spices and easily solve that problem. Sure, herbs and spices don't taste exactly like salt, but your palette will be just as happy and it won't miss the salt at all — trust us.

Here are several herbs and spices that will make you forget you ever needed a salt shaker (remove it from your table while you're at it):

- **Parsley:** You can add parsley to many dishes to give them a fresher taste and increase the flavor of other herbs and spices, like the ones in tomato sauce. A salad of lentils, beans, and parsley is a perfect Mediterranean dish. Parsley added to homemade salad dressing greatly increases the flavor of the dressing.

- **Sage:** Sage has a strong smell and a lemony, woody flavor, which lends great taste to chicken, eggs, onions, and apples. Sage goes great in bean dishes. Add it and the other herbs to soups. Sage adds delicious taste to fish or chicken when wrapped together in parchment paper.

- **Savory:** Savory is a member of the mint family and has a spicy taste similar to oregano or marjoram. Summer savory and winter savory are related, but winter savory has a stronger flavor. The name derives from the satyr, a horny goat that supposedly lives in fields of savory, and the herb has a reputation as an aphrodisiac. Worth trying, right? But some people believe it's only summer savory that has that effect. In any case, savory is great with green beans and lentils. It's good with egg dishes and adds delicious flavor to stews. Add it to green vegetables and beans. Savory alone can replace salt in your diet. It's the Herb of the Year for 2015.

- **Cilantro:** Cilantro comes from the leaves of the plant *Coriandrum sativum.* The seeds of the same plant make up coriander. Cilantro is said to have aphrodisiac properties. It brings out the flavor of other foods and can be sprinkled on cooked dishes and added to soups. Some people don't like the taste of cilantro. Decide for yourself!

- **Basil:** Basil is one of Dr. Rubin's favorite herbs. Like savory, it's a member of the mint family. It's one of the oldest herbs used in Mediterranean cooking. Needless to say, basil, too, is considered an aphrodisiac. Basil has a million uses. You can add it to tomatoes with a little olive oil; use it in pesto sauce; add it to other herbs and spices; include it in soups and stews; and use it with fish, chicken, vegetables oils, jellies, teas, and on and on.

- **Pepper:** Pepper is the "king of spices." It was the major ingredient in the European spice trade for hundreds of years. There are several colors of pepper from different stages of the same plant, but we're talking about black pepper here. The best use of black pepper is ground on to food toward the end of the cooking process because it loses its flavor and aroma if cooked too long. It can be added to almost every type of recipe.

Besides the wonderful tastes that herbs and spices add to your food, they do so with the addition of virtually no calories.

If this little discussion has whetted your appetite to start using herbs and spices, you can find enormous amounts of useful information about many more herbs and spices in *Cooking with Spices For Dummies,* by Jenna Holst (Wiley).

Switching to Whole Grains

Grains (also called cereals) are the seeds of grasses that are cultivated for foods. They come in all sizes, from popcorn to teff, a grain that is so small that when it falls on the ground it's lost. The parts of a grain include

- **Germ:** The small reproductive part of the grain, making up 3 percent of the grain by weight. The germ is rich in nutrients.

- **Endosperm:** The tissue surrounding the germ, providing nutrition for the germ, making up 83 percent of the grain by weight. The endosperm is loaded with vitamins and minerals but especially starch (carbohydrate) and protein.

- **Bran:** The hard outer layer of the grain, making up 14 percent of the grain by weight. The bran is rich in fiber.

Whole grains have all three parts. When grains are refined (milled) they lose the germ and the bran. Refining was developed to give grains a longer shelf life and better texture. White flour, for example, is all endosperm. Whole grains (not refined grains) are important sources of fiber, selenium, potassium, and magnesium. Food manufacturers enrich grains to add back some of the lost B vitamins but not the fiber.

The Mediterranean diet uses only whole grains like barley, brown rice, buckwheat, bulgur, millet, oatmeal, popcorn, whole-wheat bread, whole-wheat pasta, whole-wheat crackers, and wild rice. Here are ways to enjoy whole grains:

- Eat only the best-quality whole-grain bread from bakeries, not the supermarket, where the emphasis is on shelf life, not taste.

- Until your family enjoys whole grains, mix white and whole wheat together (for example, in pasta).

- Use some of the spices in the preceding section to add more taste.

- Use brown rice, wild rice, bulgur, and other new tastes.

- Substitute rolled oaks or crushed bran cereal for refined cereals.

- Add wild rice to soups, stews, and salads.

- Add some sweetening in the form of overripe bananas or a little honey.

Enjoying Fish or Poultry rather than Meat

Twice a week, substitute fish or poultry for meat. Yes, that means cutting out steaks, hamburgers, sausages, hot dogs, pork, and lamb. By doing this, you significantly reduce the saturated fat and cholesterol in your diet. But you don't need to lose anything in the taste of your protein source. You can use the herbs and spices described earlier to add delicious tastes to your poultry. As for fish, you have numerous choices, including the following:

- ✔ Salmon
- ✔ Tuna
- ✔ Squid
- ✔ Atlantic mackerel
- ✔ Herring
- ✔ Sardines
- ✔ Bluefish
- ✔ Rainbow trout
- ✔ Sablefish
- ✔ Pacific oysters

What these fish have in common is that they're high in omega-3 fatty acids, but so far supplements of omega-3 fatty acids haven't been shown to have the same value.

Switching to Olive Oil in Place of Animal Fat or Butter

Most of the countries that border the Mediterranean Sea, especially Spain, Italy, and Greece, grow enormous quantities of olives. When the olives are pressed, they produce olive oil. Olive oil has been eaten in the Mediterranean for more than 6,500 years. Though none of the citizens of those countries have lasted that long, men on the Greek island of Ikaria reach the age of 90 at two and a half times the rate that Americans do, and they live a decade longer free of any disease, including depression and dementia. The Ikarians' diet, like that of others around the Mediterranean, is rich in olive oil and vegetables, low in dairy (except goat's milk) and meat products, and also includes moderate amounts of alcohol. It emphasizes homegrown potatoes, beans (garbanzo, black-eyed peas, and lentils), wild greens, and locally produced goat's milk and honey.

Olive oil alone isn't responsible for the increased longevity — the whole lifestyle accounts for that — but olive oil has numerous benefits, including the following:

- ✔ It has substances that reduce inflammation, an important contributor to both cancer and diabetes.

- ✔ It prevents heart disease by lowering bad cholesterol and raising good cholesterol.

- ✔ It reduces blood pressure.

- ✔ People who consume higher levels of olive oil have less rheumatoid arthritis.

- ✔ It improves bone mineralization and calcification.

You can use olive oil in place of butter in just about any recipe. Cooking usually gets rid of the aromatic olive oil flavors. Here's how you can convert the amount of butter to olive oil:

Butter	*Olive Oil*
1 teaspoon	¾ teaspoon
1 tablespoon	2¼ teaspoons
¼ cup	3 tablespoons
⅓ cup	¼ cup
⅔ cup	½ cup
¾ cup	½ cup + 1 tablespoon
1 cup	¾ cup

Avoiding Highly Processed and Fast Foods

Highly processed and fast foods are loaded with fat and salt, and people who eat a lot of fast foods are heavier and less healthy than those who don't. Fast foods are never a part of the diet of people like those described in the previous section who live a long, healthy life. What can you do to break the fast-food habit? Here are some suggestions:

- ✔ Figure out how much you spend on fast food and begin to cut back.

- ✔ Keep a journal of why and when you eat fast food. If there are certain stimulants that promote fast-food eating, try to respond with a different behavior like exercise or cooking a delicious Mediterranean meal.

✔ Use fast-food nutrition charts to calculate all the extra calories, fat, and salt you're consuming. Start cutting back.

✔ Eliminate low-nutrition, high-calorie foods one at a time. Start with soda (including diet ones). Don't bring fast foods into your house.

✔ Replace fast food with healthy food.

✔ Make it harder to eat fast foods. Plan to walk to any fast-food restaurant, for example.

Consuming Vegetables throughout the Day

You can't eat too many vegetables. To eat a significant amount of calories through vegetables, you would have to eat so much that you wouldn't be able to eat much of anything else. That's not a bad thing.

What makes you think that you can use broccoli only as a side dish with your meat or fish? How can you possibly get in your daily three to five servings of vegetables if you think like this? What would happen if you drank vegetable juice for breakfast? Suppose you added vegetables to an omelet? How about a salad at lunch instead of that large sandwich containing way too much carbohydrate?

You can find so many different kinds of vegetables in the grocery store, but most people limit themselves to just a few of them. Your whole meal can consist of vegetables with a small amount of protein thrown in just as a garnish. Try a vegetarian restaurant to see for yourself how delicious freshly prepared vegetables can be!

We're not talking about the starchy vegetables — such as beans, peas, lentils, corn, and potatoes — that really belong in the starch list of exchanges, but rather the vegetables that contain much less carbohydrate. These vegetables include asparagus, bok choy, green beans, cabbage, carrots, cauliflower, chard, collards, onions, summer squash, turnips, and water chestnuts.

Use these vegetables in meals and for snacks. They fill you up but add very few calories. Some are just as good when frozen and defrosted as they are when fresh (because they're flash frozen immediately after picking). Especially good snack vegetables include baby carrots, cucumbers, and pieces of sweet pepper. Your cart at the market should reflect MyPlate (see Chapter 2) with an emphasis on fresh vegetables and fruits.

Avoiding High-Fat Dairy Products and Added Fat in Recipes

Food manufacturers have tried to satisfy the demand for lowfat dairy products like cheeses, cream cheese, yogurt, and sour cream. In some cases, they've succeeded. You have to try them for yourself to know just how close they come to the high fat you're used to, but the saving in kilocalories will be huge over time. Dairy is rich in calcium, potassium, and vitamin D, so it remains an important part of a complete Mediterranean diet, but unless you enjoy goat's milk, it should be lowfat or even nonfat.

If you use recipes that have been handed down in your family, they often contain a lot of unnecessary added fat. The same can be said for recipes created by chefs who aren't conscious of the harmful effects of high fat intake. We carefully selected the recipes in this book to minimize unhealthy added fat, and you should try to do the same thing when you cook.

Cooking food doesn't generally require the extra fat. Try cutting the cup of oil in your zucchini bread to ¾ cup. Although vegetable oil is better for you than animal fats like lard and butter, it still has plenty of calories — in fact, as much as animal fats. A gram of fat contains 9 kilocalories, no matter the source.

Try reducing the suggested fat by 50 percent. See whether the taste suffers or if preparing the food is more difficult.

How much difference does reducing the fat make in terms of kilocalories? A cup of oil is 8 ounces, and each ounce is 28.35 g. Because each gram has 9 kilocalories, a cup of oil contains about 2,000 kilocalories. You get rid of 1,000 kilocalories by cutting the fat in half. If your recipe serves four people, each person is getting 250 kilocalories less fat. Is that a worthwhile reduction? You bet!

Snacking on Dried Fruit or Unsalted Nuts

An apple, 4 apricots, a banana, ¾ cup blueberries, 12 cherries, 15 grapes, an orange, 1 pear, 2 plums, 1¼ cups strawberries, 1½ cups watermelon . . . all these represent just 60 kilocalories. Compare that to typical pieces of yellow cake with vanilla frosting (239 kilocalories), pound cake (116 kilocalories), pineapple upside-down cake (367 kilocalories), Boston cream pie (232 kilocalories), strawberry shortcake (428 kilocalories), or apple crumb cake (540 kilocalories). Even the cake with the fewest kilocalories has twice that of a fruit choice!

But how can you give up cakes in favor of fruits? Make it easy to eat a fruit and hard to eat cake. Don't keep cake in the house. Do keep bowls of fruit visible and in easy reach. If you must have that occasional piece of cake, don't buy a whole cake — just buy one piece and cut it in four pieces so you eat one-quarter piece each time.

Alternately, you can eat some nuts for a snack, but make sure they're unsalted and don't eat too many at a time. The following selections are about the same kilocalories as that piece of fruit:

- ✔ 6 almonds
- ✔ 1 tablespoon cashews
- ✔ 2 whole pecans
- ✔ 10 large peanuts
- ✔ 2 whole walnuts
- ✔ 2 teaspoons pumpkin seeds

This simple but profound change in your eating habits will reveal itself on the scale very rapidly. You'll be eating almost two-thirds of a pound fewer calories per week — a three-pound weight loss each month in addition to all the other changes you're making.

Sipping a Little Wine and a Lot of Water

Wine, especially red wine, is a fixture of the Mediterranean diet. But like everything else, the people of the Mediterranean area drink it in moderation. That means two 5-ounce glasses for men and one for women with a maximum of ten per week. And it's usually consumed with meals. ***Remember:*** Wine is better than beer or liquor for your health.

We don't know exactly what it is in wine that helps, but we suspect it's is the substance resveratrol. Yet taking resveratrol separate from wine doesn't seem to help. Wine in moderation reduces bad cholesterol and increases good cholesterol. So when you raise a glass "to your health," it may have some basis in fact.

Water should be your main nonalcoholic beverage. And don't waste your money on fancy bottled waters. Water is water. We're blessed in the United States with clean, clear healthy water coming out of the tap. The old rule of eight 8-ounce glasses of water a day was not based on scientific evidence. You can drink less, but it should still be your main source of liquid. Some of the main functions of water are

✔ To replace all the water you lose each day through urination, evaporation, breathing, and defecation

✔ To help you feel full so you don't eat more

✔ To maintain cleansing the body through kidney function

✔ To maintain normal bowel function

Filling Up on Legumes

Legumes include beans, peas, and lentils. They have little fat and no cholesterol, and they provide folic acid, potassium, iron, magnesium, and several other nutrients. The fats they do contain are good for you, and legumes are loaded with fiber. Their high protein content makes them a very good substitute for meat, fish, or poultry. They include black beans, black-eyed peas, chickpeas, edamame, fava beans, lentils, lima beans, kidney beans, and over 13,000 other varieties. They can be used in soups, salads, stews, as snacks, to make hummus (chickpeas), and anywhere you feel like throwing in a few legumes.

The dried legumes need to be soaked to rehydrate them before you cook them. Then you cook them in water to soften them. They can be made into dips or eaten directly as snacks. To reduce the production of intestinal gas, don't cook them in the soaking water — use canned beans or cook them very slowly.

Legumes make you feel full, a very definite benefit. If you combine legumes with whole grains, you'll be getting all nine essential amino acids, the building blocks for protein in your body. Soybeans alone have all the essential amino acids. Like berries, legumes contain lots of antioxidants, healthful substances that protect the eyes, the skin, the immune system, and the brain.

Chapter 21

Ten Keys to a Normal Blood Glucose

In *Diabetes For Dummies,* 4th Edition, we describe the management of diabetes in detail. In this chapter, you find the highlights of that extensive discussion. Although this book is about eating, controlling your blood glucose requires much more from you. Everything we suggest is directed toward normalizing your blood glucose.

Doctors consider your blood glucose *normal* when it's less than 100 mg/dl (5.5 mmol/L) if you've eaten nothing for 8 to 12 hours. If you've eaten, your blood glucose is normal if it's less than 140 mg/dl (7.8 mmol/L) two hours after eating. If you never see a blood glucose level higher than 140, you're doing very well, indeed. See Chapter 1 for a full explanation of mg/dl (milligrams per deciliter) and mmol/L (millimoles per liter).

You can use many tricks to achieve this level of control. In this chapter, you find the best of the lot. All our patients can remember receiving and using some advice that made a huge difference in their lives with diabetes. If you have a tip that you want to share, please send an e-mail to drrubin@ drrubin.com. We'll try to get it into the next edition of this book.

Knowing Your Blood Glucose

No excuse is adequate for you to not know your blood glucose at all times, although we've heard some pretty far-out excuses over the years — close to "The dog ate my glucose meter." The capability to measure blood glucose accurately and rapidly is the greatest advance in diabetes care since the discovery of insulin. Yet many people don't track their blood glucose.

Sure, sticking your finger hurts, but laser devices now make it painless, and even the needles are so fine that you barely feel them. How can you know what to do about your blood glucose if you don't know what it is in the first place?

The number of glucose meters you can choose is vast, and they're all good. Your insurance company may prefer one type of meter, or your doctor may have computer hardware and software for only one type. Other than those limitations, the choice is yours.

 If you have very stable blood glucose levels, test once a day — some days in the morning before breakfast, other days in the evening before supper. Varying the time of day you test your blood glucose gives you and your doctor a clearer picture of your control under different circumstances. If your diabetes requires insulin or is unstable, you need to test at least before meals and at bedtime in order to select your insulin dose.

Painless devices for measuring blood glucose are right around the corner. The closeness of this great advance is a particularly good reason to keep aware of new developments (see "Becoming Aware of New Developments" later in this chapter about tracking advancements).

Using Exercise to Control Your Glucose

When people are asked how much exercise they do, about a third say that they do nothing at all. If you're a person with diabetes and consider yourself a part of that group that doesn't exercise, then you aren't taking advantage of a major tool — not just for controlling your blood glucose but also for improving your physical and mental state in general. When a large group of people who were expected to develop diabetes because both parents had diabetes participated in a regular exercise program in one recent study, 80 percent who stayed on the program didn't develop diabetes.

Don't think that exercise means hours of exhaustion followed by a period of recovery. We're talking about a brisk walk, lasting no more than 60 minutes, every day, and not necessarily all at once. If you want to do more, that's fine, but most people can do this much. People who can't walk for some reason can get their exercise by moving their arms. To lose weight as a result of exercise, you need to do 90 minutes a day, every day.

Exercise can provide several benefits to your overall health. Exercise does the following:

✔ Lowers the blood glucose by using it for energy

✔ Helps with weight loss

✔ Lowers bad cholesterol and triglyceride fats and raises good cholesterol

✔ Lowers blood pressure

✔ Reduces stress levels

✔ Improves mood

✔ Reduces the need for drugs and insulin shots

When we see a new person with diabetes, we give him or her a bottle of pills. These pills aren't to be taken by mouth; they're to be spilled on the floor and picked up every day. It's our way of making sure that a new patient gets at least a little exercise every day.

Taking Your Medications

You have the advantage of having some of the best drugs for diabetes available to you, which wasn't true as recently as 15 years ago. A few years ago, as specialists in diabetes, we struggled to keep our patients in good control to avoid complications of diabetes. Now, with the right combination of medications (and by using some of the other tools in this chapter), just about any patient can achieve excellent control. But no medication works if you don't take it.

The word *compliance* applies here. Compliance refers to the willingness of people to follow instructions — specifically, taking their medications. People tend to be very compliant at the beginning of treatment, but as they improve, compliance falls off. Diabetic control falls off along with it.

The fact is, as you get older, the forces that contribute to a worsening of your blood glucose tend to get stronger. You want to do all you can to reverse that tendency. Taking your medications is an essential part of your overall program.

If you're confused by all the medications you take, get yourself a medication box that holds each day's medications in separate compartments so you make sure the compartment for each day is empty by the next day. Any doctor who prescribes more than two medicines to you should be able to get one for you, and you can definitely get them in drugstores.

Seeking Immediate Help for Foot Problems

One error that leads to a lot of grief in diabetes is failure to seek immediate help for any foot problems. Your doctor may see you and examine your feet only once in two or three months. You need to look at your feet every day. At the first sign of any skin breakdown or other abnormality (such as discoloration), you must see your doctor. In diabetes, foot problems can go from minor to major in a very brief time. We don't pull punches in this area, because seeing your doctor is so important — major problems may mean amputation of toes or more. (See Chapter 1 for more information about foot problems as they relate to diabetes.)

You can reverse most foot problems, if you catch and treat them early. You may require a different shoe or need to keep weight off the foot for a time — minor inconveniences compared to an amputation.

Besides inspecting your feet daily, here are some other actions you can take:

- Testing bath water with your hands to check its temperature, because numb feet can't sense if the water is scalding hot

- Ensuring that nothing is inside your shoe before you put it on

- Wearing new shoes only a short time before checking for damage

Taking immediate action goes for any infection you develop as a diabetic. Infections raise the blood glucose while you're sick. Try to avoid taking steroids for anything if you possibly can. Steroids really make the glucose shoot up.

Brushing Off Dental Problems

Keeping your teeth in excellent condition is important, but especially if you have diabetes. "Excellent condition" means brushing them twice a day and using dental floss at the end of the day to reach where the toothbrush never goes. It also means visits to the dentist on a regular basis for cleaning and examination.

We have seen many people with diabetes have dental problems as a result of poor dental hygiene. As a side effect, controlling the blood glucose is much harder. After patients cure their teeth, they require much less medication.

People with diabetes don't have more cavities than non-diabetics, but they do have more gum disease if their glucose isn't under control. Gum disease results from the high glucose that bathes the mouth — a perfect medium for bacteria. Keeping your glucose under control helps you avoid losing teeth as a result of gum disease, as well as the further deterioration in glucose control.

Maintaining a Positive Attitude

Your mental approach to your diabetes plays a major role in determining your success in controlling the disease. Think of diabetes as a challenge — like high school math or asking out your first date. As you overcome challenges in one area of your life, the skills you master help you in other areas. Looking at something as a challenge allows you to use all your creativity.

When you approach something with pessimism and negativity, you tend to not see all the possible ways you can succeed. You may take the attitude that "It doesn't matter what I do." That attitude leads to failure to take medications, failure to eat properly, failure to exercise, and so forth.

Simply understanding the workings of your body, which comes with treating your diabetes, probably makes you healthier than the couch potato who understands little more than the most recent sitcom.

Some people do get depressed when they find out they have diabetes. If you're depressed and your depression isn't improving after several weeks, consider seeking professional help.

Planning for the Unexpected

Life is full of surprises — like when you were told you have diabetes. You probably weren't ready to hear that news. But you can make yourself ready to deal with surprises that may damage your glucose control.

Most of those surprises have to do with food. You may be offered the wrong kind of food, too much food, or too little food, or the timing of food doesn't correspond to the requirements of your medication. You need to have plans for all these situations before they occur.

You can always reduce your portions when the food is the wrong kind or excessive, and you can carry portable calories (like glucose tablets) when food is insufficient or delayed.

Other surprises have to do with your medication, like leaving it in your luggage — which is on its way to Europe while you're headed to Hawaii. Keep your important medications with you in your carry-on luggage, not in checked luggage. Again, your ability to think ahead can prevent you from ever being separated from your medication.

Not everything is going to go right all the time. However, you can minimize the damage by planning ahead.

Becoming Aware of New Developments

The pace of new discoveries in diabetes is so rapid that keeping on top of the field is difficult even for us, the experts. How much more difficult must it be for you? You don't have access to all the publications, the drug company representatives, and the medical journals that we see every day.

However, you can keep current in a number of ways. The following tips can help you stay up-to-date on all the advances:

- Begin by taking a course in diabetes from a certified diabetes educator. Such a course gives you a basis for a future understanding of advances in diabetes. The American Diabetes Association (www.diabetes.org) provides the names of certified diabetes educators.

- Get a copy of Dr. Rubin's book *Diabetes For Dummies,* 4th Edition (Wiley), which explains every aspect of diabetes for the nonprofessional.

- Join a diabetes organization, particularly the American Diabetes Association. You'll start to receive the association's excellent publication, *Diabetes Forecast,* in the mail, which often contains the cutting edge of diabetes research as well as available treatments.

- Go to Dr. Rubin's website (www.drrubin.com), where you can find linkable addresses for the best and latest information about diabetes on the Net.

- Finally, don't hesitate to question your doctor or ask to see a diabetes specialist if your doctor's answers don't satisfy you.

The cure for diabetes may be in next week's newspaper. Give yourself every opportunity to find and understand it.

Utilizing the Experts

The available knowledge about diabetes is huge and growing rapidly. Fortunately, you can turn to multiple people for help. Take advantage of them all at one time or another, including the following people:

- Your primary physician, who takes care of diabetes and all your other medical concerns

- A diabetes specialist, who is aware of the latest and greatest in diabetes treatment

✔ An eye doctor, who must examine you at least once a year

✔ A foot doctor, to trim your toenails and treat foot problems

✔ A dietitian, to help you plan your nutritional program

✔ A diabetes educator, to teach you a basic understanding of this disease

✔ A pharmacist, who can help you understand your medications

✔ A mental health worker, if you run into adjustment problems

Take advantage of any or all of these people when you need them. Most insurance companies are enlightened enough to pay for them if you use them.

Avoiding What Doesn't Work

Not wasting your time and money on worthless treatments is important. When you consider the almost 20 million people with diabetes in the United States alone, they provide a huge potential market for people with "the latest wonder cure for diabetes." Before you waste your money, check out the claims of these crooks with your diabetes experts.

You can find plenty of treatments for diabetes on the Internet. One way you can be sure that the claims are based on science is to look for verification from the Health on the Net Foundation, which you can find at www.hon.ch/HomePage/Home-Page.html. Its stamp of approval means the site adheres to principles that every legitimate scientist agrees with.

Don't make any substantial changes in your diabetes management without first discussing them with your physician.

Chapter 22

Ten Strategies for Teaching Kids Healthy Eating Habits

Children don't hate vegetables any more than they hate ice cream. It is what we teach them that determines their feelings about food. If we show them that we love vegetables and consider them delicious, that's how they will feel about vegetables. They love to follow our example. The best time to do this is at family meals.

Fruit is no problem. Try taking a bowl of sweet strawberries, blueberries, or raspberries away from a small child! It's not quite as dangerous as taking a bone from a dog, but close. Most children have a natural love for sweet. There is nothing like a sweet peach or nectarine to excite a child. Just try to get ripe fruit, not the too-early-picked, hard-as-a-rock, tart stuff that passes for fruit in many markets.

There are numerous things you can do to encourage your child to eat vegetables. In this chapter, we provide just ten. We're sure you can come up with a few others.

One thing we don't encourage is this idea of concealing the vegetables from the child. The message you send is that vegetables are so unpleasant that you have to fool the child to get him to eat them, exactly the message that will lead to a life of avoiding vegetables.

Starting Early

Children learn their eating habits at a very young age, age 2 or even younger. From the time they can eat solid or even semi-solid food, they should be given choices of vegetables. We do not recommend using bottled vegetables, since they are often filled with salt and sugar, but rather making the vegetables into small portions yourself.

Give the child the vegetable to eat by itself, not with a choice of fatty things or sweet things that he will gravitate towards. Do not threaten that the "good stuff" comes only after the vegetables are eaten. Vegetables must be seen as part of the good stuff.

And, of course, set an example. Let him see you eating and enjoying the vegetables. The message will come through loud and clear.

Letting Children Pick

Children love to feel that they have power. Give them the power to pick the vegetables in the market that they and you will eat. Move around to the different colors, explaining that the reason for the different colors is that each color represents a different kind of food that they need in their body. Get a rainbow of vegetables.

Try to know what the vegetables contain so you can explain to the child. Much of that information is in Chapter 2. This vegetable gives you this vitamin and mineral. That vegetable gives you that one. Your body uses them all to create a healthy person.

Involving Children in Food Preparation

When you ask children to describe their earliest memories, they often talk happily about helping their grandmother make some kind of food. Many of the chefs in this book began cooking by their grandmother's or mother's side.

Preparing food together can be a great bonding experience between you and your child, and it also provides you with the opportunity to teach good nutrition. If your child helps you to prepare vegetables, he will want to try what he has prepared.

Have your child create his or her own nutrition plan for a day and discuss every part of it, pointing out what is carbohydrate, protein, fat, the balance among those foods, and how they affect his or her diabetes. Use MyPlate (www.choosemyplate.gov) or the child's nutrition plan as a guide for planning, showing the important role that vegetables play in the plan.

Never prepare one meal for your diabetic child and another for the rest of the family. Everyone can benefit from the better choices you make with your child's nutritious food. The child also realizes that eating isn't punishment for a person with diabetes because the whole family eats the same way.

Keeping Problem Foods Out of Sight and Good Foods in Easy View

If potato chips or creamy cookies sit on the kitchen counter, can you blame your child (or yourself) for grabbing a handful every time he or she goes by? Don't buy these foods in the first place. If you do, keep them out of sight. You know what happens when you walk up to a buffet table. You can more easily avoid what you don't see.

On the other hand, keep fruits and vegetables in plain sight. Have carrot sticks and celery sticks easily available. Keep some cooked broccoli and cauliflower in the refrigerator.

Again, your child follows your example. If you raid the freezer for ice cream, don't be surprised to see your child do the same thing. If you raid the refrigerator for broccoli or asparagus, that is what your child will do as well. The great benefit to you when you set an example for your child is the excellent nutrition that you get.

Growing a Garden

Even if all you have is a small box, you can show your child where vegetables come from, how they grow, when to pick them, and the fun of eating what you grow. Plus, foods that you grow and pick yourself, just at the peak of taste, are a totally different experience from what you get at the market. Only the farmer's market can come close. So if you can't possibly grow your own, take your child to a farmer's market. They are everywhere.

If you do have a little space, here are a few recommendations from an old farmer (Dr. Rubin). Grow some bush beans from seeds for the beautiful flowers that precede the delicious and plentiful beans, and to demonstrate what can come from a tiny seed. They don't require staking up like pole beans. Grow some beets and carrots, also from seeds, to show that foods grow under the earth as well as above the earth, and they get pretty sweet at that. Grow some tomatoes and zucchini from plants to show how things can grow in abundance from only one or two plants that start very tiny.

Dr. Rubin invited his friends' grandchildren, who live in a big city, to see his garden. He pulled a carrot out of the earth and offered it to the 3-year-old. He looked at it and said, "Next time, put pieces of carrot in the earth to make it easier for eating." Since he had only seen pieces of carrot in the past, he thought that was how they grew.

Let your child do the picking. The thrill of picking your own food is not to be missed. If you can't pick in your own garden, pick where you can pay for the produce in another garden.

Finding Vegetable Recipes They Like

In the age of the Internet, the availability of great recipes is almost overwhelming. In this book, you find a tiny portion of what is out there. Brilliant chefs are working to produce recipes that make us salivate. Your children will love the results.

Appendix D has our recommendations for sources for great recipes, not just for people with diabetes, but for everyone. One of the central themes in all our books about diabetes is that people with diabetes can eat great food. They can eat just about anything as long as the portions are appropriate.

You don't have to go to vegetarian sources to find great vegetable recipes. Even restaurants that feature meat know how to cook vegetables. You'll be amazed at the creative ways that chefs prepare zucchini, carrots, squash, spinach, and so forth.

Try watching some of the cooking shows on TV as you exercise. Check the schedule and try to exercise when the vegetable cooking is being shown. The only problem is that you may want to stop exercising and start cooking. Resist until you have done your 30 minutes or more.

Stir-Frying

One of the best ways to cook vegetables ending with a delicious dish without adding a lot of fat is to stir-fry. You use very little oil and the vegetables come out hot and delicious. The natural tastes of the vegetables are sealed in. The Chinese have been doing it this way for generations. Until they adopted our Western styles of cooking and eating, diabetes was not much of a problem among the Chinese.

Stir-fry many different kinds of vegetables together to make a vegetable medley. Some may take a little longer or a little shorter to fry so put the ones together that take the same time. A meal made up just with stir-fried vegetables can be all your child needs to realize how delicious vegetables can be. You don't have to throw in any chicken or beef. That is an important message to send your child. A meal can be complete without animal protein. As we've emphasized in past editions, eating vegetarian is a very healthful way to go.

Using a Dip

Sometimes dipping the vegetables into a delicious dip that you prepare can make the vegetables even more delicious, desirable, and easy to eat. Here is a simple dill dip mix that your child will love:

- ½ cup dried dill weed
- ½ cup dried minced onion
- ½ cup dried parsley
- ½ cup Beau Monde seasoning

Combine the ingredients in a bowl and store in a tight container. Label it with instructions for use. When needed, combine 1 cup lowfat mayonnaise, 1 cup lowfat yogurt, and 3 tablespoons of dill dip mix and blend well. Your child will love it with all vegetables.

Knowing the Right Sized Portion

A 2-year-old child requires a lot less than a 20-year old adult. The recommended serving size of vegetables for a toddler is a tablespoon per year of age. If you want to get your 2-year-old to eat five of his servings of vegetables, all you have to do is get him to eat ten tablespoons during the course of the day. That's a lot easier than you thought. If your child wants more, don't stop him!

With so little that has to be eaten to reach the daily goal, it may be easier to stick to just one or two vegetables on any given day. Today is carrot and bean day while tomorrow is beet and zucchini day. Vegetables can be fun!

Giving Fruit Juice

You would never think of offering your child a cigarette, would you? Why would you ever offer your child a can of soda? Chapter 2 makes it pretty clear that there is little difference in the negative consequences of cigarettes or soda or fruit drinks, for that matter. If you want to get some more fruit into your child and he won't eat enough solid fruit, give him 100 percent fruit juice. You can get juice from just about any fruit and many vegetables.

You can also make delicious fruit smoothies with lots of fruit, some juice, and a little yogurt. Kids love them!

Don't buy the canned variety, which always has too much salt in it for some dumb reason. Get a juicer and make your own. The wonderful possibilities of putting together all kinds of fruit flavors is easily available if you make your own. Connect the drinking of juice with some kind of celebration. In Dr. Rubin's house they have juice with breakfast every morning and clink their glasses together as they say, "To life!"

Part V
Appendixes

Nutrition Facts
Serving Size 1/2 cup (113g)
Servings Per Container 4

Amount Per Serving

Calories 120   Calories from Fat 15

% Daily Value

Total Fat 1.5g	3%
Saturated Fat 1.0g	5%
Cholesterol 10mg	3%
Sodium 290mg	12%
Total Carbohydrate 15g	5%
Dietary Fiber 0g	
Sugars 14g	
Protein 10g	10%

For *Dummies* can help you get started with lots of subjects. Visit www.dummies.com to learn more and do more with *For Dummies*.

In this part . . .

- ✔ Find the restaurants that provided the great recipes throughout this book.
- ✔ Learn the language of cooking, from al dente to zest.
- ✔ Convert ounces to grams, Fahrenheit to Celsius, and more.
- ✔ Find sources for more recipes in books and online.

Appendix A

Restaurant Descriptions

· ·

*A*fter you've had a chance to look over and try some of the wonderful dishes in this book, you'll never again think that people with diabetes can't enjoy terrific meals! The chefs who contributed these recipes are health- and nutrition-conscious, and you'll probably be able to find other choices on their menus that also fit your nutritional plan very well. However, note that we've tried to reduce kilocalories by reducing fat and sugar intake as much as possible — with the agreement of the chefs — as well as by keeping salt intake on the low side.

The meal you receive in the restaurant may not be *exactly* what you find here, especially because chefs change often; also, chefs sometimes cook for 100 or more people, and their measurements may not be exact every time. Most food must be prepared rapidly in a restaurant and not the same way. You'll also receive a portion that is generally too large, so be prepared to take some home.

The restaurants that contributed recipes for this book are all fine restaurants that have been given the stamp of approval by various testing organizations. You won't be disappointed no matter what you eat in these establishments, but the kilocalories and the distribution of carbohydrate, protein, and fat may not fit your nutritional plan perfectly. You need to adjust other meals and snacks to get your overall nutrition plan to conform to the guidelines for a full day (see Chapter 2).

The difficulty of preparation for the recipes in this book varies greatly. For a few reasons, we include some recipes that are more labor-intensive and time-intensive than usual:

- ✔ You may be an excellent cook and willing to try these recipes despite the time and work involved, because they're delicious and worth the effort.

- ✔ Even if you choose not to try specific recipes, you'll find wonderful tips about foods and techniques to incorporate into whatever you cook.

- ✔ You'll get an idea of what goes into the magical foods that these fine restaurants are turning out, and you can choose to order that dish if you go to that restaurant.

Whatever your pleasure, *bon appétit!*

Restaurant Descriptions

The following sections introduce the restaurants in this book and the recipes they contributed. Each establishment offers innovative cuisine and a quality dining atmosphere.

AltaMare Restaurant

1233 Lincoln Rd., Miami Beach (phone: 305-532-3061; web: `www.altamare restaurant.com`)

AltaMare is a favorite with Miami South Beach locals and features beautifully presented fresh fish and classic Italian cuisine. Chef Claudio Giordano and his wife, Kaituska, work their magic with phenomenal seafood, fresh pasta, and tasty soups served in a decor that reflects South Beach style. These aspects come together in a menu that showcases the best catches from local fishing boats and wonderful Italian dishes. Chef Giordano has been awarded the North American Restaurant Association Award of Excellence for two years in a row.

AltaMare has provided the following recipes:

- ✔ AltaMare Fish Soup (Chapter 12)
- ✔ Fettuccini Shrimp (Chapter 12)
- ✔ Grouper Acquapazza (Chapter 12)

Barbetta

321 W. 46th St., New York City (phone: 212-246-9171; web: `www.barbetta restaurant.com`)

Barbetta, the oldest restaurant in New York, still run by its founding family, recently celebrated its 100th birthday. In addition, it is the oldest Italian restaurant in New York and the oldest restaurant in New York's Theater District. It was started in 1906 by Sebastiano Maioglio, the father of the current owner, Laura Maioglio. Laura has transformed her restaurant into New York's first truly elegant Italian dining destination. Good nutrition is important to Laura Maioglio. She has added new recipes to the current edition and the following recipes from Barbetta confirm her focus on health:

- ✔ Fresh Jumbo Lump Crabmeat with Wild Rice Sautéed in Sherry (Chapter 12)
- ✔ Fresh Mushroom Salad (Chapter 9)

🖛 Granita of Lemon (Chapter 16)

🖛 Paillard of Chicken Breast with Fennel and Parmigiano (Chapter 13)

🖛 Pears Baked in Red Wine alla Piemontese (Chapter 16)

🖛 Risotto alle Erbe Made with Extra-Virgin Olive Oil (Chapter 10)

🖛 Salad of Imported Mozzarella di Bufala, Cherry Stem Tomatoes, and Fresh Basil (Chapter 9)

Candle 79, Candle Cafe East, and Candle Cafe West

Three locations: 154 E. 79th St., New York City (phone: 212-537-7179; web: www.candle79.com); 1307 Third Ave., New York City (phone: 212-472-0970; web: www.candlecafe.com/east); and 2427 Broadway, New York City (phone: 212-769-8900; web: www.candlecafe.com/west)

Candle Cafe serves local, organic, vegan food. It was started in 1984 by Bart Potenza who was joined in 1987 by Joy Pierson. Their food is dedicated to good health, using vegetables and fruits grown without pesticides and other chemicals. Their work together has led to the *Candle Cafe Cookbook, Candle 79 Cookbook, Vegan Holiday Cooking,* and a national line of vegan frozen foods.

They provided the following recipes:

🖛 Cucumber and Avocado Soup (Chapter 8)

🖛 Roasted Root Vegetables and Quinoa (Chapter 10)

Cetrella

845 Main St., Half Moon Bay, California (phone: 650-726-4090; web: www.cetrella.com)

Lewis Rossman, the executive chef at Cetrella, has rapidly turned this fine restaurant into a destination. The menu features elegantly rustic northern Mediterranean cuisine inspired by the coastal villages of France, Italy, and Spain. Lewis emphasizes using the local produce, cheeses from nearby artisans, and seafood from the nearby Pacific Ocean. These are the recipes that Lewis Rossman has kindly provided for our readers:

🖛 Rock Shrimp Ceviche (Chapter 12)

🖛 Vegetable Fritto Misto (Chapter 11)

David Burke Townhouse

133 E. 61st St., New York City (phone: 212-813-2121; web: www.davidburke townhouse.com)

David Burke Townhouse features the cuisine of one of America's fastest rising young chefs, David Burke. He has received numerous other awards for his fine cuisine. David's training was at the Culinary Institute of America in Hyde Park, New York. Following that, he served in a number of great restaurants in the United States and went to France to fine-tune his skills. David's genius with fresh ingredients keeps his restaurant filled every night with VIPs and others. The restaurant provided the following recipe:

✔ Zucchini and Cucumber Linguine with Clams (Chapter 11)

Hangawi

12 Park Ave., New York City (phone: 212-213-1001; web: www.hangawi restaurant.com)

Hangawi's owners, William and Terri Choi, started the restaurant 15 years ago because they believe vegetarianism is the healthiest diet. They translated many of their favorite Korean dishes for Western vegetarians. They use many ingredients that they bring back from Korea to produce food for which their restaurant has been voted the best vegetarian restaurant in New York. Hangawi provided the following recipe:

✔ Organic Tofu and Shiitake Mushrooms (Chapter 11)

Kanella

1001 Spruce St., Philadelphia (phone: 215-922-1773; web: www.kanella restaurant.com)

Konstantinos Pitsillides makes "fabulous things happen" in the kitchen of his "homelike" Greek-Cypriot restaurant in Washington Square West, Philadelphia. He creates fantastic fresh seafood that pleases the palate and satisfies foodies. The place is down to earth, and what you see is what you get. The service is attentive and efficient. Sundays they offer a great-value meze prix fixe.

Kanella contributed the following recipes:

✔ Cyprus Bulgur Wheat Salad (Chapter 10)

✔ Gigante Beans (Chapter 11)

The Lark

6430 Farmington Rd., West Bloomfield, Michigan (phone: 248-661-4466; web: www.thelark.com)

The Lark is a sophisticated European-style country inn located in the heart of West Bloomfield, Michigan. The award-winning cuisine is prepared with French cooking techniques. Chef Kyle Ketchum was trained at several fine restaurants after graduating from Le Cordon Bleu of Scottsdale, Arizona. He combines the finest local ingredients with his special skills to produce food that has consistently won awards, including *Bon Appétit* magazine's "One of America's 10 Best Special Occasion Restaurants" and *Condé Nast Traveler* magazine's "Best Restaurant in the United States."

Chef Kyle Ketchum from The Lark provided the following recipes:

- Cantaloupe-Papaya Salad with Ginger Simple Syrup (Chapter 16)
- Goat-Cheese-Stuffed Zucchini with Yellow Tomato Sauce (Chapter 11)
- Seared Diver Scallops with Bacon and Shallot Reduction (Chapter 12)
- Watermelon Gazpacho (Chapter 8)

Millennium

580 Geary St., San Francisco (phone: 415-345-3900; web: www.millennium restaurant.com)

Millennium chef Eric Tucker and owner Ann Wheat have created a gourmet dining experience of vegetarian, healthy, and environmentally friendly foods. Many cultures are responsible for the delicious flavors and styles you will find there.

Millennium has provided the following recipes:

- Baby Artichokes, Gigante Beans, and Summer Vegetable Cartoccio with Cream Polenta (Chapter 11)
- Quinoa and Black Bean Salad over Chilled Avocado Soup (Chapter 10)
- Vietnamese-Style Stuffed Grape Leaves (Chapter 11)

The Olive and Grape

8516 Greenwood Ave. N., Seattle (phone: 206-724-0272; web: www.theolive andgrape.com)

This lovely restaurant marries Turkish and Mediterranean specialties such as chicken kabob, hummus, and moussaka. The owner, Paola Corsini, draws on her Italian, Greek, and Turkish heritage to create dishes that bring a unique blend of flavors to the wonderful food served at this neighborhood favorite. The restaurant features imported Turkish olive oils and the freshest ingredients from the Pacific Northwest. And to top it all off, there is delicious homemade baklava and gelato!

The Olive and Grape has kindly provided the following recipes:

- ✔ Arugula Salad (Chapter 9)
- ✔ Turkish Meatball Kofte (Chapter 14)

Paley's Place

1204 NW 21st Ave., Portland, Oregon (phone: 503-243-2403; web: `www.paleysplace.net`)

Vitaly Paley, chef of Paley's Place, was born near Kiev in the former Soviet Union. He studied at the French Culinary Institute in New York and fine-tuned his skills at fine restaurants in New York and France. Vitaly came to Portland and opened Paley's Place with his wife, Kimberly, in 1995.

The cuisine is French bistro fare. The ingredients are from the Pacific Northwest from local farmers and ranches. Vitaly uses them to produce classic food similar to the classic music he once performed. Paley's Place contributed the following recipes to this book:

- ✔ B.B.Q. Cedar-Planked Salmon (Chapter 12)
- ✔ Summer Tomato Salad (Chapter 9)
- ✔ Truffle Vinaigrette (Chapter 9)

Poggio

777 Bridgeway, Sausalito, California (phone: 415-332-7771; web: `www.poggiotrattoria.com`)

Poggio is the dream of famed restaurateur Larry Mindel, who has been creating great restaurants for 30 years. Past creations include Ciao and Prego in San Francisco; Guaymas in Tiburon, California; and MacArthur Park in San Francisco and Palo Alto. He also pioneered the concept of the Italian bakery and restaurant at Il Forniao. He has been recognized by the Italian government for his contribution to preserving the Italian heritage outside of Italy.

Larry is joined in the kitchen by chef and partner Chris Fernandez. At Poggio he uses the best of the local ingredients to make classic Italian food with care and respect.

Poggio provided these recipes for this book:

- ✔ Red-Wine-Braised Lentils (Chapter 10)
- ✔ Spinach-Ricotta Gnocchi (Chapter 15)

Rathbun's

112 Krog St., Ste. R, Atlanta (phone: 404-524-8280; web: www.rathbuns restaurant.com/dinner-menu.html)

Rathbun's is the dream of executive chef Kevin Rathbun, who developed his great love for extraordinary food at a very young age. Kevin began in restaurants as an apprentice at age 14. Soon he was working for such famous chefs as Bradley Ogden and Emeril Lagasse at Commander's Palace in New Orleans. In 2004, Kevin opened Rathbun's, where he features a Modern American menu. Aware of the problems of obesity, Kevin offers small plates for those who limit their portions. Rathbun's contributed the following recipes for this book:

- ✔ Cauliflower-Parmesan Soup (Chapter 8)
- ✔ Pan-Roasted Cod with Shrimp and Mirliton Squash (Chapter 12)
- ✔ Pan-Roasted Veal Chops with Corn and Gouda Ragoût (Chapter 14)
- ✔ Zucchini and Parmigiano-Reggiano Salad (Chapter 11)

Revival Bar and Kitchen and Venus Restaurant

2102 Shattuck Ave., Berkeley, California (phone: 510-549-9950; web: www.revivalbarandkitchen.com); 2327 Shattuck Ave., Berkeley, California (phone: 510-540-5950; web: www.venusrestaurant.net)

Amy Murray is the founder and visionary of multiple successful East Bay eateries, including Revival Bar and Kitchen and Venus Restaurant. Amy started her first local, organic, seasonal restaurant in 1994, as a young pioneer of this movement in the East Bay. She was inspired by the small village food model of most of the nonindustrial world as she traveled around 17 Asian countries in the early 1990s. Amy dedicated herself to this movement to bring cleaner, healthier, nontoxic food, grown without chemicals, to provide more culinary vitality to the people.

Revival is proud to refer to itself as Berkeley's own local food shed, complete with artisan cocktails, handmade delicacies from local growers, happy charcuterie, and thoughtfully prepared California food in a revived 1901 classic building. Snout to tail, root to shoot, Revival offers local, organic, and dynamic food, sourced from local food sheds from within 100 miles. It features whole animal butchery from grass-fed animals, which are carefully raised in nearby Marin.

Venus opened in 2000 as one of the first casual, small-farm, organic eateries in Berkeley and has a loyal following of fans who enjoy the NorCal-style brunch and dinner menus.

Amy offered the following recipes:

- Chawan Mushi Egg Custard and Clams (Chapter 12)
- Chili Lime Mint Vinaigrette Watermelon Salad (Chapter 9)
- Gluten-Free Skillet Cornbread (Chapter 10)
- Pickled Sardine Appetizer (Chapter 7)
- Swordfish with Lemon Salsa (Chapter 12)

Sublime

1431 N. Federal Hwy., Fort Lauderdale (phone: 954-539-9000; web: `www.sublimerestaurant.com`)

Sublime is the vision of owner Nanci Alexander, who wanted to show that plant-based food could be sublime. It has an award-winning menu featuring natural and organic foods and spirits from around the globe. The cuisine has received numerous awards.

Sublime has provided the following:

- Brown Rice Pudding (Chapter 16)
- Tuscan Quiche (Chapter 6)

Suze Restaurant

4345 W. Northwest Hwy., Dallas (phone: 214-350-6135; web: `www.suzedallas.com`)

Suze Restaurant is one of the best in Dallas. It has been recognized by *Bon Appétit,* the *Zagat Guide,* and *USA Today* and is renowned for its fine food, extensive wine list, neighborhood appeal, and cozy atmosphere. Executive Chef Gilbert Garza's menus feature a unique mix of classic dishes and seasonal specialties. The restaurant uses fresh produce, meat, and dairy from local farmers and trusted vendors.

Chef Garza kindly provided these recipes:

- ✔ Egg Salad with Hummus (Chapter 9)
- ✔ Grilled Summer Chicken Tartare (Chapter 13)
- ✔ West African Braised Chicken (Chapter 13)

Tante Marie's Cooking School

271 Francisco St., San Francisco (phone: 415-788-6699; web: www. tantemarie.com)

Tante Marie's Cooking School was founded in 1979 by Mary Risley to provide all-day, year-round classes for people who want to cook well. She has been the recipient of "Cooking Teacher of the Year" and "Humanitarian of the Year." The school covers all cuisines. Its graduates serve as chefs, food writers, cooking teachers, pastry chefs, and caterers. Tante Marie's has provided a number of vegetarian recipes for this book, but you can learn whatever cuisine you are interested in at their school.

Tante Marie's has provided the following recipes:

- ✔ Asparagus Bread Pudding Layered with Fontina (Chapter 11)
- ✔ Asparagus Pizza with Fontina and Truffle Oil (Chapter 11)
- ✔ Cacit (Cucumber Dip) (Chapter 7)
- ✔ Fig, Mozzarella, and Mizuna Salad with Thai Basil (Chapter 9)
- ✔ Heirloom Tomato Soup with Fresh Basil (Chapter 8)
- ✔ Omelet with Wild Mushrooms (Chapter 6)
- ✔ Portobello Mushroom Sandwich (Chapter 11)
- ✔ Tante Marie's Muesli (Chapter 15)
- ✔ Vegetable Frittata (Chapter 6)

A City-by-City Restaurant Travel Guide

So that you can use this section as a kind of travel guide, we've listed the restaurants by cities, in alphabetical order.

Atlanta

Rathbun's

Dallas

Suze Restaurant

Miami–Fort Lauderdale

AltaMare Restaurant

Sublime

New York City

Barbetta

Candle 79

Candle Cafe East

Candle Cafe West

David Burke Townhouse

Hangawi

Philadelphia

Kanella

Portland, Oregon

Paley's Place

San Francisco Bay Area

Cetrella

Millennium

Poggio

Revival Bar and Kitchen

Tante Marie's Cooking School

Venus Restaurant

Seattle

The Olive and Grape

West Bloomfield, Michigan

The Lark

Appendix B

Glossary of Key Cooking Terms

• •

al dente: Cook to slightly underdone with a chewy texture, usually applied to pasta.

bake: Cook with hot, dry air.

barbecue: Cook on a grill, using charcoal or wood.

baste: Spoon melted butter, fat, or other liquid over food.

beat: Mix solid or liquid food thoroughly with a spoon, fork, whip, or electric beater.

bind: Add an ingredient to hold the other ingredients together.

blanch: Plunge food into boiling water until it has softened, to bring out the color and loosen the skin.

blend: Mix foods together less vigorously than beating, usually with a fork, spoon, or spatula.

boil: Heat liquid until it rolls and bubbles.

bone: Remove the bone from meat, fish, or poultry.

braise: Brown foods in fat and then cook slowly in a covered casserole dish.

bread: Coat with bread crumbs.

broil: Cook by exposing directly to high heat.

brown: Cook quickly so the outside of the food is brown and the juices are sealed in.

caramelize: Dissolve sugar and water slowly and then heat until the food turns brown.

ceviche: Placing raw seafood in an acid to "cook."

chop: Cut food into small to large pieces.

curdle: Cause separation by heating egg- or cream-based liquids too quickly.

deglaze: Pour liquid into a pan of meat — after roasting or sautéing and after removal of fat — to capture the cooking juices.

degrease: Remove fat from the surface of hot liquids.

devein: Remove the dark brownish-black vein that runs down the back of a shrimp.

dice: Cut into cubes the size of dice.

dilute: Make a liquid, such as a sauce, less strong by adding water.

drain: Remove liquid by dripping through a strainer.

drippings: The juice left after meat is removed from a pan.

dry steaming: Cooking foods such as vegetables in their own natural juices rather than adding additional moisture.

dust: Sprinkle lightly with sugar or flour.

emulsify: Bind hard-to-combine ingredients, such as water and oil.

fillet: Cut meat, chicken, or fish away from the bone.

fold: Mix together without breaking.

fry: Cook in hot fat over high heat until brown.

fumet: A heavily concentrated stock.

garnish: Decorate food.

grate: Shred food in a grater or food processor.

grease: Lightly cover a pan with fat to prevent food from sticking.

grill: Cook on a rack over hot coals or under a broiler.

hors d'oeuvres: Bite-sized foods served before dinner.

infusion: Extract flavor from a food into a hot liquid.

julienne: Cut vegetables and other foods into matchstick-sized strips.

knead: Work dough to make it smooth and elastic.

leaven: Cause to rise before and during baking.

marinate: Place in a seasoned liquid to tenderize.

meringue: Egg whites beaten with sugar and baked.

mince: Chop food very fine.

pan-roast: A two-step process that first sears and seals a thicker piece of meat or chicken in a pan on the stovetop and then finishes that piece in the oven, in the same pan you started with.

pan-broil: Cook on top of the stove over high heat, pouring off fat or liquid as it forms.

parboil: Partially cook food in boiling water.

pare: Remove skin from a fruit or vegetable.

phyllo: A tissue-thin layer of dough.

pickle: Preserve food by submerging in a salty brine.

pilaf: A rice dish seasoned with herbs and spices, combined with nuts, dried fruits, poultry, and vegetables.

pinch: The amount of food you can take between two fingers.

poach: Submerge food in a liquid that is barely boiling.

proof: Test yeast — to find out whether it's active — by mixing with warm water and sugar.

puree: Break food into small particles (examples are applesauce and mashed potatoes).

reduce: Boil down a liquid to concentrate the taste of its contents.

roast: Cook in dry heat.

sauté: Brown food in very hot fat.

sear: Subject foods such as meat to extremely high heat for a short period of time to seal in juices.

shred: Tear or cut into very small, thin pieces.

simmer: Cook over low heat, never boiling.

soufflé: A baked food made light by egg whites.

steam: Cook food over a small amount of boiling water.

steep: Place dry ingredients in hot liquid to flavor the liquid (tea is an example).

stew: Slowly cook meat and vegetables in liquid in a covered pan.

stir-fry: Quickly cook meat or vegetables in a wok with a little oil.

stock: A liquid in which solid ingredients (like chicken meat and bones, vegetables, and spices) are cooked and then usually strained out.

sweat: Cook over low heat in a small amount of fat (usually butter) to draw out juices to remove rawness and develop flavor.

toast: Brown by baking.

vinaigrette: A dressing of oil, vinegar, salt, pepper, and various herbs and spices.

whip: Beat rapidly to add air and lighten.

zest: The outermost colored peel of an orange or other citrus fruit that is cut, scraped, or grated to add flavor to foods.

Appendix C

Conversion Guide

. . . .

Do you know how many tablespoons are in a cup? How many grams are in a pound? And how do you choose between all those sugar substitutes on the market? What if you need to convert an oven temperature from Celsius to Fahrenheit? This appendix offers some information to help you answer those questions.

Conversions

The following list provides some common measurement conversions.

> 1 teaspoon = ⅓ tablespoon
>
> 1 tablespoon = 3 teaspoons
>
> 2 tablespoons = ⅛ cup (1 ounce)
>
> 4 tablespoons = ¼ cup
>
> 5⅓ tablespoons = ⅓ cup
>
> 8 tablespoons = ½ cup
>
> 16 tablespoons = 1 cup
>
> 1 cup = ½ pint
>
> 2 cups = 1 pint
>
> 2 pints = 1 quart
>
> 4 quarts = 1 gallon
>
> 1 pound = 16 ounces
>
> 1 fluid ounce = 2 tablespoons
>
> 16 fluid ounces = 1 pint

Table C-1 explains how to convert specific measurements. For example, if you have 3 *ounces* of mushrooms, how many *grams* of mushrooms do you have? To find out, multiply 3 by 28.35 (you have 85.05 grams).

Table C-1	Conversion Methods	
To Convert	*Multiply*	*By*
Ounces to grams	Ounces	28.35
Grams to ounces (dry)	Grams	0.035
Ounces (liquid) to milliliters	Ounces	30.00
Cups to liters	Cups	0.24
Liters to U.S. quarts	Liters	0.95
U.S. quarts to liters	Quarts	1.057
Inches to centimeters	Inches	2.54
Centimeters to inches	Centimeters	0.39
Pounds to grams	Pounds	453.59

Table C-2 shows you the differences between Fahrenheit and Celsius temperatures.

Table C-2	Temperature (Degrees)
Fahrenheit	*Celsius*
32	0
212	100
250	120
275	140
300	150
325	160
350	180
375	190
400	200
425	220
450	230
475	240
500	260

Sugar Substitutes

The new approach to nutrition for people with diabetes doesn't emphasize the elimination of sugar from your diet entirely as long as you count the kilocalories that you consume. When a recipe calls for only a few teaspoons of sugar, you may want to use table sugar (also known as *sucrose*). When the recipe calls for ¼ cup of sugar or more, then substitution with a noncaloric sweetener of your choice will definitely save you kilocalories. There are also sweeteners besides glucose that do contain kilocalories but offer other advantages, such as not raising the blood glucose as fast. (We discuss your sweet options in more detail in Chapter 2.)

The following sweeteners contain kilocalories that are added into the total kilocalorie count. They're absorbed differently than glucose, so they affect the blood glucose differently.

- Fructose, found in fruits and berries
- Xylitol, found in strawberries and raspberries
- Sorbitol and mannitol, sugar alcohols occurring in plants

Non-nutritive or artificial sweeteners are often much sweeter than table sugar. Therefore, much less of this type of sweetener is required to accomplish the same level of sweetness as sugar. The current artificial sweeteners (from oldest to newest) include the following:

- Acesulfame-K (such as Sunett)
- Aspartame (such as NutraSweet)
- Saccharin (such as Sweet'N Low)
- Stevia (such as Truvia)
- Sucralose (such as Splenda)

If you plan to substitute another sweetener for sugar, check out Table C-3 to find the measurements needed to achieve equal sweetness.

Table C-3		Sweetener Equivalents			
Sugar	*Fructose*	*Acesulfame-K*	*Aspartame*	*Saccharin*	*Sucralose*
2 teaspoons	⅔ teaspoon	1 packet	1 packet	⅛ teaspoon	1 packet
1 tablespoon	1 teaspoon	1¼ packets	1½ packets	⅓ teaspoon	1½ packets
¼ cup	4 teaspoons	3 packets	6 packets	3 packets	6 packets
⅓ cup	5⅓ teaspoons	4 packets	8 packets	4 packets	8 packets
½ cup	8 teaspoons	6 packets	12 packets	6 packets	12 packets
⅔ cup	3½ tablespoons	8 packets	16 packets	8 packets	16 packets
¾ cup	¼ cup	9 packets	18 packets	9 packets	18 packets
1 cup	⅓ cup	12 packets	24 packets	12 packets	24 packets

Appendix D

Other Recipe Sources for People with Diabetes

· ·

So many cookbook recipes are available for people with diabetes that this book wouldn't have been written if it didn't offer a special feature, namely the recipes of some of the finest chefs in the United States. In this appendix, we provide a list of excellent Mediterranean cookbooks, as well as the best of the vegetarian cookbooks in case you don't eat meat.

You can find even more recipes online. You can generally count on the recipes in books to contain the nutrients they list, but online recipes may not be as reliable; you need to evaluate the site before accepting the recipes. You can trust the sites that we list here. You can find them by typing the address into your web browser.

Cookbooks for People with Diabetes

No book like this one exists on cooking for people with diabetes. Those listed in this section offer recipes for home-grown meals, not the creative work of great chefs. However, plenty of useful information and tons of good recipes appear in the books we list here.

- *Healthy Mediterranean Cooking,* by Rena Salaman (Frances Lincoln)
- *How to Cook Everything Vegetarian: Simple Meatless Recipes for Great Food,* by Mark Bittman (Houghton Mifflin Harcourt)
- *Meatless: More Than 200 of the Very Best Vegetarian Recipes,* by Martha Stewart Living (Clarkson Potter)
- *The Mediterranean Diet,* by Marissa Cloutier and Eve Adamson (Harper)
- *The Mediterranean Diet Cookbook: A Mediterranean Cookbook with 150 Healthy Mediterranean Diet Recipes* (Rockridge University Press)

- *Mediterranean Diet Cookbook For Dummies,* by Meri Raffetto, RD, and Wendy Jo Peterson, MS, RD (Wiley)

- *The Mediterranean Diet for Beginners: The Complete Guide* (Rockridge University Press)

- *Mediterranean Diet For Dummies,* by Rachel Berman, RD (Wiley)

- *The Mediterranean Diet for Every Day: 4 Weeks of Recipes & Meal Plans to Lose Weight* (Telamon Press)

- *The Mediterranean Diet: Unlock the Mediterranean Secrets to Health and Weight Loss with Easy and Delicious Recipes,* by John Chatham (Rockridge University Press)

- *Mediterranean Harvest: Vegetarian Recipes from the World's Healthiest Cuisine,* by Martha Rose Shulman (Rodale Books)

- *The Mediterranean Heart Diet: Why It Works, With Recipes to Get You Started,* by Helen V. Fisher with Cynthia Thomson, PhD, RD (De Capo Press)

- *The Mediterranean Prescription: Meal Plans and Recipes to Help You Stay Slim and Healthy for the Rest of Your Life,* by Angelo Acquista, MD (Ballantine Books)

- *The Mediterranean Vegan Kitchen,* by Donna Klein (HP Trade)

- *Mediterranean Women Stay Slim, Too: Eating to Be Sexy, Fit and Fabulous,* by Melissa Kelly with Eve Adamson (William Morrow)

- *My New Mediterranean Diet: Eat Better, Live Longer by Following the Mediterranean Diet,* by Jeannette Seaver (Arcade Publishing)

- *The New Mediterranean Diet Cookbook: A Delicious Alternative for Lifelong Health,* by Nancy Harmon Jenkins (Bantam)

- *The New Vegetarian Cooking for Everyone,* by Deborah Madison (Ten Speed Press)

- *The Oh She Glows Cookbook: Over 100 Vegan Recipes to Glow from the Inside Out,* by Angela Liddon (Avery Trade)

- *The Oldways 4-Week Mediterranean Diet Menu Plan: Make Every Day Mediterranean* (Oldways)

- *The Southern Vegetarian Cookbook: 100 Down-Home Recipes for the Modern Table,* by Justin Fox Burks and Amy Lawrence (Thomas Nelson)

- *Vegetarian Cooking For Dummies,* by Suzanne Havala, MS, RD (Wiley)

Food and Recipe Websites for People with Diabetes

In this section, we list our favorite online resources for Mediterranean and vegetarian recipes. Keep checking back at these websites. They're constantly adding new recipes.

- ✔ **101 Cookbooks:** www.101cookbooks.com/vegetarian_recipes

- ✔ **Allrecipes.com: Mediterranean Diet:** www.allrecipes.com/recipes/healthy-recipes/special-diets/mediterranean-diet

- ✔ **Allrecipes.com: Vegetarian Recipes:** www.allrecipes.com/recipes/everyday-cooking/vegetarian

- ✔ **Cooking Light: Superfast Mediterranean Recipes:** www.cookinglight.com/food/quick-healthy/superfast-mediterranean-dishes-20-minutes-or-less

- ✔ **Cooking Light: Vegetarian:** www.cookinglight.com/food/vegetarian

- ✔ **Eating Well:** www.eatingwell.com/recipes_menus/collections/healthy_mediterranean_recipes

- ✔ **Epicurious.com:** www.epicurious.com/recipesmenus/global/mediterranean/recipes

- ✔ **Food Network: Healthy Mediterranean:** www.foodnetwork.com/healthy/packages/healthy-mediterranean.html

- ✔ **Food Network: Vegetarian Recipes:** www.foodnetwork.com/topics/vegetarian-recipes.html

- ✔ **Vegetarian Times:** www.vegetariantimes.com/recipe

Index

About the Authors

Alan L. Rubin, MD, is one of the nation's foremost experts on diabetes. He is a professional member of the American Diabetes Association and the Endocrine Society and has been in private practice specializing in diabetes and thyroid disease for over 40 years. Dr. Rubin was assistant clinical professor of medicine at University of California Medical Center in San Francisco for 20 years. He has spoken about diabetes to professional medical audiences and nonmedical audiences around the world. He has been a consultant to many pharmaceutical companies and companies that make diabetes products.

Dr. Rubin was one of the first specialists in his field to recognize the significance of patient self-testing of blood glucose, the major advance in diabetes care since the advent of insulin. As a result, he has been on numerous radio and television programs, talking about the cause, prevention, and treatment of diabetes and its complications. His first book, *Diabetes For Dummies,* now in a fourth edition, is a basic reference for any nonprofessional who wants to understand diabetes. It has sold more than 1 million copies and has been translated into 19 languages including French, Chinese, Spanish, and Russian. He is also the author of *Thyroid For Dummies, High Blood Pressure For Dummies, Type 1 Diabetes For Dummies, Prediabetes For Dummies,* and *Vitamin D For Dummies* (all published by Wiley).

Cait L. James, MS, has overseen health education programs at Kaiser Permanente and counseled clients in individualized nutrition and personal fitness plans in health clubs over the past 15 years. After receiving her undergraduate degree in Journalism and Health from the University of Oregon, she earned a Master of Science degree in Health Education focused on the prevention and treatment of obesity. This led her to Kaiser Permanente's Pediatric Clinic, working with children suffering from or at risk of medical complications due to weight. While this grew into the oversight of a wide variety of health promotion programs for patients and staff, the promotion of healthy nutrition choices continues to be her biggest passion. She loves great food and wine, so thankfully she balances it with avid running and yoga!

Dedication

This book is dedicated to the great chefs and restaurant owners, especially the ones in this book, who spend all their time and creative energy producing delicious and nutritious food in a beautiful environment and making sure that it is served in a way that complements the taste.

Authors' Acknowledgments

Acquisitions editor Tracy Boggier, who shepherded this fourth edition through all the committees that had to approve it, deserves special commendation. Our project editor, Elizabeth Kuball, made certain that the book is understandable and readable in the great *For Dummies* tradition.

Heather Dismore is responsible for most of the discussions of food and the organization of the recipes in the book, and she also contributed a number of excellent recipes. Her tremendous skill in doing so is apparent in this book and in another book that she helped author, *Cooking Around the World All-in-One For Dummies*.

Special thanks to Dr. Rubin's wife, Enid, who spent hours on the phone and the computer gathering new recipes that featured the Mediterranean philosophy of cooking and providing the food and comfort that allowed Dr. Rubin to complete this book.

Denise Sharf is also responsible for many of the classic recipes that have remained in the book throughout all its editions.

Reviewers Rachel Nix and Emily Nolan did a fantastic job of ensuring that the information in the book is accurate.

Publisher's Acknowledgments

Senior Acquisitions Editor: Tracy Boggier

Project Editor: Elizabeth Kuball

Copy Editor: Elizabeth Kuball

Technical Editor: Rachel Nix

Recipe Tester: Emily Nolan

Art Coordinator: Alicia B. South

Project Coordinator: Emily Benford

Photographer: T. J. Hines

Cover Image: © iStock.com/tsartsianidis